PRAISE FOR *Lives Reimagined: Changing the Course of Psychotic Illness*

"Should be required reading for anyone who wants to help a person with neuropsychiatric brain disease (NBD). Truly a beacon of hope, as promised, in what can seem like a bleak landscape. A guiding light for those diagnosed with NBD, the practitioners who guide their recovery, and the families and friends who love them. Thank you for actionable ideas, heartfelt stories, and caring so much about people like my son. Finally we can reimagine life—again."

—**Randye Kaye**, Author, *Ben Behind His Voices;*
Podcast Host, *Schizophrenia: 3 Moms in the Trenches*

"Severe mental illness ranks with cancer as one of the two most terrifying and destructive scourges known to mankind—corrosive and incurable. From the founding of the barbaric Bedlam Asylum in London eight centuries ago to the criminally rudderless care and treatment of "crazy people" today, fear, ignorance, bumbling and neglect have hobbled progress in combatting the affliction.

Breakthroughs in microcomputer technology in the 1980s allowed scientists to see severe mental illness for what it is: not a metaphor for unhappiness, but a palpable, organic failure in brain cells. Amidst the growing literature springing from this discovery, *Lives Reimagined: Changing the Course of Psychotic Illness* is the latest and among the best. Co-authors Lisa Mann, PhD and Katharine Cutts Dougherty, PhD, have produced a rich and far-ranging compendium of fact, interpretation, advice, and medical insights that shed powerful light on what is now called "neuropsychiatric brain disease" and an "unfolding road map" for the general reader seeking enlightenment. This book, seminal in its aims and comprehensive in its flow of information and ideas, is destined to become a standard."

—**Ron Powers**, Pulitzer-Prize winning journalist;
Author, *No-one Cares About Crazy People*

"Both my family and I are eternally grateful to have been mentored by and privileged to collaborate with the greats of psychiatry. We started with the esteemed Deborah Levy, PhD, and then came Lewis Opler, MD, PhD and E. Fuller Torrey, MD. The culmination of our journey through the rough seas of neuropsychiatric brain disease (NBD) has brought us to the welcoming calm harbor of Rocco Marotta MD, PhD. What we have all learned together is that there is a correct approach to NBD. Simply put, build embracing relationships with your patients and families, use the most effective treatments as early as possible (clozapine based), and be eternally patient. Most importantly dare to hope. The Lodge experience and the Team Daniel experience both show meaningful recovery is not only possible, but it is probable if appropriate resources are made available. Lisa's and Katharine's loving treatise is a demonstration of how far kindness and competence can take you on this journey. Read, learn and be enlightened."

—**Rob Laitman, MD** and **Ann Mandel Laitman, MD**,
Co-Authors, *Meaningful Recovery from Schizophrenia and Serious Mental Illness with Clozapine*

"This compelling account of Dr. Rocco Marotta's clinical program for psychosis at Silver Hill Hospital serves as both a sobering reminder of the ongoing crisis—where high-THC cannabis is harming the developing brains of vulnerable young people—and a hopeful testament to the power of evidence-based, compassionate care. By integrating the strengths of therapeutic community, psychotherapy, and medication, this program offers a model for healing. Professionals, parents, and policymakers alike should read this book to grasp the urgent challenges before us and the promising path forward."

—**Patrick Kennedy**, Co-Founder, *The Kennedy Forum*

Lives Reimagined
Changing the Course of Psychotic Illness

Lisa Mann, PhD
Katharine Cutts Dougherty, PhD

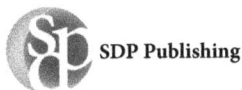

SDP Publishing

Lives Reimagined, published July, 2025
Editorial and proofreading services: Kent Sorsky; Beth Raps; Gina Sartirana
Interior layout and cover design: Howard Johnson
Photo credits: Front cover image owned by Katharine Cutts Dougherty

SDP Publishing

Published by SDP Publishing, an imprint of SDP Publishing Solutions, LLC.

To obtain permission(s) to use material from this work, please submit an email request with subject line: SDP Publishing Permissions Department, to: info@ SDPPublishing.com.

ISBN-13 (print): 979-8-9922388-1-5

ISBN-13 (ebook): 979-8-9922388-2-2

Library of Congress Control Number: 2025907221

This book is dedicated to the individuals who struggle with neuropsychiatric brain disease, their families, and the professionals who seek to help and support them.

TABLE OF CONTENTS

PREFACE

If you are reading this book, chances are that serious mental illness—or, as we prefer, neuropsychiatric brain disease (NBD)—has touched you or the life of someone you love or with whom you work closely. You may have boarded multiple vessels in your attempt to arrive at that elusive destination of sustained mental health, navigating often frustrating and occasionally enraging mental health rules and regulations. Some of you have had to be both captain and crew for your journey. It is easy to feel overwhelmed, confused, and lonely in the struggle to keep going.

Lives Reimagined: Changing the Course of Psychotic Illness is a guiding lifeline and a beacon of hope for those struggling to help loved ones submerged by their vulnerability to disruptive psychotic episodes. It describes the transformative approach of The Lodge acute care program (one of the residential programs at Silver Hill Hospital in New Canaan, Connecticut), which has helped countless patients reimagine and attain a meaningful life. Developed and directed by Dr. Rocco Marotta, known for his enduring impact on patients and families, the founding premise of the program is that individuals struggling with neuropsychiatric brain disease should not be defined by their illness but rather should be helped to live lives filled with connection to family, friends, and a sense of meaning. The Lodge team's measure of successful outcomes goes beyond reduction of acute psychotic symptoms to rebuilding sustained stability, agency, and purpose.

This book describes the stabilizing elements that support long-term success and will help families and providers recognize when an unstable vessel threatens to disrupt their loved one's ability to thrive. Each chapter of the book discusses a different aspect of this unique program, providing the reader with a specific approach to the diagnosis and treatment of neuropsychiatric illness. Critically, the end of each chapter presents con-

cepts and key elements that can be used by readers to develop more successful goals and treatment interventions for the loved ones in their care.
Through descriptions of the program, interwoven with personal stories
from Lodge program alums and their families, and interviews with team
members, readers will come to understand The Lodge team's view of the
core components of sustained stability, and gain valuable information
that can help them negotiate the myriad issues that threaten to untether
loved ones from their lifelines. Navigating neuropsychiatric brain disease
can be exhausting. While you may not access this particular program,
we hope this book will help you feel less alone and fill you with a sense of
possibility.

Each of the authors has had a unique window to the work that is
described. As Rocky's senior research associate, Katharine has spent five
years sitting in Rocky's office with him several times a week, watching
him in patient, family, and staff meetings, and helping him further his
research interests in this field, preparing papers, presentations, and case
conferences. As Rocky's wife and a trained clinical psychologist, Lisa has
collaborated with him for many years on developing presentations and
colloquiums, and has participated in decades of parent advisory groups
and case discussions.

In writing this book, Lisa and Katharine have interviewed many of
the current and former staff at The Lodge, along with colleagues of Rocky
from other institutions, and reached out to some of Rocky's patients and
their parents, offering them the opportunity to contribute to this book.
Anyone quoted in this book has given informed consent for their ano-
nymized input to be included and has been given the chance to revoke
consent after reading the finished manuscript. All the personal stories
("Lived Stories") included have been quoted verbatim, without correction or editing. Finally, Rocky and Lisa have spent countless hours at the
kitchen table in what can only be described as a never-ending interview
about his work.

A Note from Katharine

There is a reason that many of us who are connected to neuropsychiatric
brain disease identify with being called warriors. As caregivers, family

members, professionals, advocates, or fellow sufferers, we are constantly on a battlefield, fighting against a wretched, poorly understood disease that threatens to destroy and wreak havoc in its path. On any given day the battlefield can change and there really is no choice but to carry on in our shared struggle for restoration and peace.

And while this book is about hope, the battle against neuropsychiatric brain disease is often lost. The greatest loss is in the people who are killed in its vicious path and those whose brains are destroyed by this disease. Then, of course, there are the families and communities whose lives are devastated by the collateral damage. The seriously mentally ill are often left to suffer on our streets or in our prisons. Unlike other diseases that destroy a single individual, neuropsychiatric brain disease casts a wider shadow and engulfs the individual first, before moving on to threaten families, communities, and whole societies. We ignore neuropsychiatric brain disease at our peril.

Bringing this book together was, in part, a mission to portray the brave efforts of the dedicated, skilled, and compassionate clinical team at The Lodge program. This team partners with families and patients, continuing to win impossible battles and to bring hope and healing. For the few stories that we have been able to share in these pages, there are countless others that remain untold. Parents often choose to preserve the confidentiality of their loved ones, particularly as the battles rage on; likewise, patients may not be willing or able to share their journeys. We therefore treasure and appreciate the stories that have been shared in this book, and we treat them as sacred.

Yet the Lodge program, as described in these pages, cannot be explained without acknowledging the pivotal role of its creator and leader, Dr. Rocco Marotta. For the past twelve years, staff have gravitated toward Rocky. He is beloved and revered by all who have had the privilege to work with him. When someone new is told to find him, it is always amusing to watch their bewilderment as they encounter him for the first time. Often, they will arrive in a timely fashion to his office, only to find Rocky already heavily engaged in conversation with someone else. "Come in," Rocky will say, and gesture to them to sit down while he proceeds with an entirely different meeting. Rocky's cell phone will ring, and he will let it continue clanging away; his office phone will ring, and he will ignore that, too. Waiting, the guest can't help but look around the cluttered office with papers strewn everywhere. Finally, Rocky will turn to them. As soon as they start talking, he will query their accent, inviting them to guess his own origins. If the guest is willing to suspend all judgment, engage in the moment, absorb the messiness, the interruptions, and the chaos that are integral to the work that happens in the world of neuropsychiatric brain disease, they soon realize that they are in the presence of an eccentric genius, a mad scientist, and an incomparable healer.

As his senior research associate, I've sat watching Rocky with patients, families, and his clinical team over the past several years. I've seen him take the hand of every patient into his own, staring into their souls and connecting with them while restoring their sense of worth and importance, giving them hope where most have failed. I've seen him as he meets with family members and addresses their concerns with honesty and urgency, picking up the phone and returning all calls to get them the resources and connections they need. Recently, I witnessed how Rocky masterfully helped someone who was literally falling asleep in his office to open his eyes, agree to a medication change, and to get labs done—all the while holding the hand of another family member in distress, and writing a new prescription. I've seen Rocky drop everything to help a fellow colleague or pause a team meeting to help everyone feel supported and regroup and refocus on the important work at hand. And finally, I've seen the deep contentment that arises when Rocky relaxes in his chair, puts his arms around his stomach, and lets out a big sigh, smiling from ear to ear. In his presentations, he describes these as his Buddha moments, similar to what is sometimes achieved through the use of oxytocin for those with NBD. For Rocky, that deep peace is achieved as he witnesses a patient begin to reemerge and connect to the world after years of hard-fought battles and suffering. Rocky truly is The Healer.

Rocky's unique leadership style and example has led many of the team to say that what he does is not science but art; that what Rocky does transcends the material and moves toward the spiritual. *"Teme Jesu,"* Rocky will often say to a patient or family, a reference to the fact that you need to be careful that you don't encounter the truth right in front of you and yet fail to see it. There is one truth, however, that Rocky's entire team, his patients, and their families have all come to know and appreciate through the years: we have been unimaginably blessed to have Rocky in our lives. Rocky has repeatedly taught us to believe in the impossible and to work together—as patients, families, and providers—to help restore hope and bring healing through unwavering love, dedication, and perseverance.

A NOTE FROM LISA

Katharine's words need no elaboration. They bear witness to the journey of those struggling with neuropsychiatric brain disease, to the work taking place in The Lodge program, and to the remarkable man who leads The Lodge team. To my mind there is not much to add except an additional personal note. I came to the writing and collaboration on this book as a parent, a psychologist, and Rocky's wife. This multidimensional perspective has allowed me to see things both from the inside out and the outside in. I am so moved by Katharine's description of the battles we face, and the need for everyday resilience in this lifelong journey, because I have lived it. I laugh out loud each time I read her description of Rocky's messy office and his eccentric brilliance, because believe me, I have lived that too!

My own personal experience with inspired teamwork actually comes from my early life as the daughter of the founder and first violinist of the Juilliard String Quartet. My father was described throughout his career as an inspiring leader, and while his technique sometimes defied the more conventional rules of pedagogy, his charisma, vision, and unmitigated passion for the art of music indelibly shaped the character of the Juilliard String Quartet during the fifty-one years he sat in the first violin chair. My father was very clear to anyone who asked, however, about his role within the quartet. Although he acknowledged and appreciated their nod to his leadership, he consistently told people it was the dynamics of all the players and the dialogue among their separate voices that created a totality that was greater than the sum of its parts. The Juilliard String Quartet was known for playing fast tempos and taking musical risks. My father would coach students, "Life is not always beautiful, not every phrase should be sweet. Don't be afraid to take risks but *listen* to what you are playing. Speak the music, breathe the music, always think about what you want to say." In so many ways, I think this describes Rocky, his Lodge team, and the work that they do.

There is no doubt that Rocky's vision and leadership have been central to The Lodge team's success. His desire to bring all to the metaphorical table, his attention to the intermingling of voices and the dynamics and morale of the team help it to become more than the sum of its parts. As one of the team members reminds us, however, great leaders don't just help their followers; they inspire and mentor others to rise to their best selves. This certainly occurs in The Lodge program.

Rocky would also be the first to remind us that there are other professionals out there who are thinking passionately about these issues, who value dialogue and listen well. They are not always easy to find, nor is it simple in our world to find a safe place in which the treatment of NBD can happen. We struggle, often, with the unfairness of this truth. But, while each of the stories so generously shared in this book are singular, they also send a universal message: **persist!** Dealing with neuropsychiatric brain disease is a life-long journey with many stops along the way. Find your allies and support one another. Search for providers who are skilled at navigating the treacherous sea of NBD, who will stay open to new ideas, and who, above all, understand the power of relationships and enduring connections in the service of changing lives. The work taking place at The Lodge is a lesson for us all. Lives challenged by NBD can be reimagined and effectively changed. Even on the darkest days, there is always room for hope.

AN IMPORTANT NOTE ABOUT TERMINOLOGY

NEUROPSYCHIATRIC BRAIN DISEASE (NBD)

As we bring you on board this journey with us, let us pause and reflect on something that will permeate every word of this book. We're talking about how we *define* the work that is being done. Specifically, we want to draw a line at the outset that we believe should be drawn systematically in this field: we want to shift from talking about "mental health" and "mental illness" to a focus on "brain health" and "brain illness." What is powerful about this shift is the ability to bring psychiatric brain illness to its rightful place alongside other physical illnesses, and in so doing, evoke greater awareness and understanding of how it can be treated and managed most successfully.

We started writing this manuscript with an acceptance of the commonly used umbrella term "serious mental illness" to capture our book's focus on individuals suffering from severe brain disease. And yet, as we found ourselves repeatedly emphasizing that psychotic disorders are *biological* diseases, we now feel compelled to insist on a new term, less entangled with stereotypes and stigma: "neuropsychiatric brain disease."

Using the term "mental" to describe neuropsychiatric brain illness immediately conjures up archetypes, philosophies, and entire religious frameworks that confuse disorders of the brain with free will and moral agency. These associations are extremely harmful and dangerous to those afflicted with brain disease. It is striking to think of all the organizations and institutions that use the term "mental health" that are actually focused on addressing brain illness.

We believe that if we had continued to use the term "mental illness" in this book, we would have been perpetuating a misconception that needs to be corrected. Neuropsychiatric disorders are biologically based and need to be treated as we would any other severe disease in the body. Appropriately labeled, "neuropsychiatric brain disease" directs us to pay attention to the underlying neurochemical processes that need to be addressed and stabilized. It also demands that insurance companies give parity to NBD with all other serious medical illnesses. Finally, the term "neuropsychiatric brain disease" offers deeper clarity for those afflicted (and their families) to understand that, just like with other chronic illnesses such as diabetes, thyroid disease, and heart disease, stability will always be dependent on treatment adherence. "Stability" is a key word here and raises another important point of distinction: having a chronic illness does not equate to living a life limited and defined by disability.

When you search for "brain health" or "brain illness" online, it is striking to note that these terms are used mainly to refer to Alzheimer's Disease. And if one looks at the World Health Organization's dedicated site on brain health, the focus is on an array of afflictions—autism, cardiovascular diseases, dementia, epilepsy, Guillain–Barré syndrome, migraine and other headache disorders, Japanese encephalitis, meningitis, Parkinson's disease, spinal cord injury, tetanus, Zika virus—with no mention of schizophrenia spectrum disorders, despite the fact that they account for a far larger proportion than many of the aforementioned diseases. Similarly, when you look at the US Center for Disease Control's main website, the focus on brain health and brain disease is entirely devoted to the aging brain or environmental or physical assaults to otherwise healthy brains, without a mention of organic brain diseases, which are found on the page that describes mental health. This is a mistake.

Language has both an obvious and subtle impact on our beliefs and experiences. Reframing neuropsychiatric disorders as neuropsychiatric brain disease (NBD) instead of serious mental illness (SMI) has implications for how patients see and accept ongoing treatment, how insurance companies view these illnesses, and how society and the legal system treat those who struggle with these diseases.

To those who are concerned that this focus on biology distracts from the psychological and social components of these illnesses, we respond that an awareness of the integration of biological, social, and emotional factors is important in *all* disease states. A thorough examination of cardiac illness, for example, involves not only an investigation of the physiology of arteries but also of stress levels and eating patterns. Similarly, we believe that using the term "neuropsychiatric brain disease" does not diminish the importance of the psychological but rather reminds us not to forget the biological. Thus, throughout this book we use the term NBD rather than SMI to denote the brain diseases that result in persistent psychotic states. We believe it is well past time for others to do so as well.

REBUILDING LIVES

We also feel it is important to define what we mean by "rebuilding lives," a phrase that we use throughout the book to denote a patient's movement toward sustained stabilization, greater agency, and increased social connection. The patients who attend The Lodge program have failed to find a stable path in life. Their lives have been repeatedly interrupted by recurring psychotic destabilization and the revolving door of psychiatric hospitalizations. Simply put, they have been trapped by their illness. The Lodge treatment program is a layered approach, where stabilization of acute symptoms is only the beginning. Over time, with processes described in detail in this book, residents of this program are able to move into a life that promises more long-term stability, connection to others, and the development of a sense of agency. We think of this as rebuilding a life torn apart by the ravages of poorly treated NBD. The bias of this book is clear: while there are many factors involved in the treatment of NBD, we believe that medication plays a critical role.

We have also consciously refrained from using the phrase "successful recovery" when discussing our patients' movement toward healthier, more integrated functioning. While someone struggling with NBD can recover from states of psychosis and dysregulation that have interrupted their ability to develop a meaningful life, they must come to accept that they are never free from this chronic illness. Accepting they have a chronic illness, however, is not incompatible with building a happy and meaningful life. Coming to this understanding is perhaps the greatest challenge for anyone living with NBD.

Introduction:
Unfolding the Map

"The person I am today is completely different from who I was....
I've accomplished things, inside and out, my old self would
think impossible.... Most of all, I see myself as someone who
has a right to live in this world."

—Alum, The Lodge program

We all know that the mental health system in the United States is broken. In the introduction to his book *Healing: Our Path from Mental Illness to Mental Health*, Thomas Insel, MD, former director of the National Institute for Mental Health, makes an honest and important statement:

> I should have been able to help us bend the curves for death and disability [in the field of mental health], but I didn't. Because ... the problem I was solving by supporting brilliant scientists and dedicated clinicians was not the problem that faced nearly fifteen million Americans living with serious mental illness.... Our science was looking for causes and mechanisms [of mental illness] while the effects of these disorders were playing out in increasing death and disability [of individuals struggling with these diseases], increasing incarceration and homelessness, and increasing frustration and despair for both patients and families.[1]

It has been the unfortunate experience of the vast majority of the parents and their children attending The Lodge program at Silver Hill Hospital in New Canaan, Connecticut, as well as so many others, that this statement is accurate. In 2022, 3.7 million Americans 18 years and older, were identified as having a lifetime history of schizophrenia spectrum disorders[2]—a group of disorders characterized by distortions of thinking, perception, and emotional expression and experience, as well as cognitive problems—and yet there are still comparatively few programs dedicated to the sustained wellness of the people who suffer from them. Even rarer are hospital programs dedicated to the goal of sustained recovery and the attainment of meaningful reconnection of patients to family, friends, and community. While millions of dollars have supported research into the underlying mechanisms of severe neuropsychiatric disease, there has been little shift in the problematic, business-oriented models of treatment which leave patients and their families traveling the same inadequate treatment paths over and over again. Too often individuals and families spend years trying to find help for their loved ones. Young people spend years of their lives in and out of hospitals and outpatient systems and are compelled to place Band-Aids on gaping wounds, leading to fragmented treatment that does not arrest the progression of the illness.

Unquestionably, there are serious issues with inequality of health-care treatment and questions that must be answered about racial differences in rates and treatment of psychotic illness.[3] The scope of this book is on an individual program which, due to its patient population, cannot address the systematic aspect of these important issues. But the risk of addiction, homelessness, and death, because of inadequate care for those struggling with neuropsychiatric brain disease, crosses socioeconomic, cultural, and racial lines. Add into the equation the legal challenges of dealing successfully with NBD, and you have a situation which can be, quite simply, devastating for any family and catastrophic for some.

It doesn't have to be that way. This book tells the story of a program and its leader who challenge the system with enormous success. Most of our readers will never have a family member attend this program, and in fact the leadership of the program itself has evolved since the writing of this book. Nonetheless, the program's results stand as a testament to the importance of challenging the standard treatment of neuropsychiatric brain disease. This book presents the unique characters of The Lodge program, but also the universal truths embodied in their approach to the work. By the end of this book, we hope there will be lessons learned and useful questions shared that you can apply to what we know can be extremely complex realities.

Dr. Rocco Marotta developed The Lodge program in response to the crisis of inadequate mental health treatment for neuropsychiatric brain disease. It is not a scientific research project, nor a neuropsychiatric research model trying to answer a few distinct questions. It is focused entirely on the actual lived experiences of up to fourteen patients at a time and their families, most of whom have been failed by previous treatments and are struggling to navigate this disease. Its focus is on the treatment of acute-phase psychotic illness and building a foundation for meaningful post-hospital life. Patterns of intervention are individualized, based on ongoing evaluation, continuing psychosocial interventions, and the use of specific and highly titrated medications. Working diagnoses are frequently revisited, and overt control of symptomatology is seen by the staff as only the first point in each individual's return to a more meaningful life. Integration into family, school, work, sports, and other aspects of more social experience is the end game. Many medication regimens are considered, used, and constantly reevaluated for effectiveness. Each medication regime is a recipe, a "secret sauce," which is created for each individual patient. Among these, clozapine*, in conjunction with oxytocin**, has proven to be a powerful tool for change in many of the most impaired individuals.

We at The Lodge program have often remarked that the story of a patient's progress is similar to that of a voyage in a vessel, navigated by a captain and a crew. We think this maritime metaphor provides a useful structure for the book.

The staff, a.k.a. "the crew," at The Lodge, are not politicians or celebrity personalities. They, and their counterparts in diverse clinical settings, are the soldiers who work the front lines of actual patient care. They are the people who have dedicated their time and experience to changing the lives of actual patients and their families, moment by moment, one life at a time. The origins of this book began with their observations and discussions. A surprising number of patients were getting remarkably better on a unique combination of medications and extended stay care. Not just remarkably better in terms of sustained reduction of positive symptoms (such as hallucinations, delusions, and distortions in thinking), but remarkably better in terms of regaining social/emotional connection to family, friends, and the world around them. Many of these patients had been placed on the neuropeptide hormone oxytocin, which Dr. Marotta, a.k.a. "the Captain," was using, along with clozapine, to combat negative symptoms*** associated with persistent psychotic illness. First it was one

---

* Clozapine is an antipsychotic medication with particular efficacy in treating resistant psychosis.

** Oxytocin is a neuropeptide hormone which impacts interpersonal relatedness, motivation, and mood regulation.

*** Negative symptoms include emotional and social withdrawal, which themselves include lack of emotional expression or feeling, difficulties with social interaction, and lack of motivation or engagement.

patient, then it was a couple, then it was such a significant number that it couldn't be coincidental. The Lodge, a.k.a. "the vessel," houses a program that involves far more than one medication or one intervention. It is about seeking the best combination of interventions for each specific individual struggling with neuropsychiatric brain disease and extending this intervention into their post-hospital life.

The clinical work, a.k.a. "the voyage," that takes place at The Lodge addresses issues from both a cognitive and relational perspective. Individuals struggling with psychotic illness have often lost a sense of who they are or want to be because their life narrative has become so modified and fractured. Distortions of thinking and emotional experience are so overwhelming that there is a tendency to equate self with symptoms (e.g., "I am bipolar" versus "I have bipolar illness") rather than other aspects of one's life experience. Extended time in a supported setting allows psychotic symptoms to subside and a more workable narrative about themselves and their life to develop. Once the haze of disorganized and distorted thinking, and the accompanying inability to process information and form connections recedes, the development of trusting relationships with the team gives each patient consistent feedback and a sense of being grounded. Extended interactions with peers also promote a sense of belonging and help them absorb different perspectives and life lessons. At The Lodge, the benefit of both these elements are seen every day.

Approaching each patient's disorder as a constellation of symptoms rather than a single diagnostic entity helps The Lodge patients to differentiate symptoms they have from the self that they are. Understanding that anxiety, for example, is due to increased heart rate gives them a sense of potential control over overwhelming experiences and a way to reframe their narratives about themselves. Prioritizing the relationship between the patient, staff, families, and other patients in their treatment interventions, and often extending outreach to patients beyond their hospital stay, reflects again and again the staff's belief that besides medication, sustained connection to others is the single most important factor in long-term stability.

The Lodge program challenges the current status quo and, unlike important scientific investigations which are many steps away from application, the lessons learned from The Lodge program are well within our grasp to implement. Unequal access to this kind of treatment saddens and enrages both those who are struggling with NBD and those who are dedicated to treating it. So does the fact that in a field of medicine where approximately fifty percent of patients are treatment-resistant, clinicians are constantly fighting with insurance companies to gain approval for the time, diagnostic procedures, and tests they need to truly do their job. If a hospital stay needs to be long enough for an extensive diagnostic evaluation to take place, an initial treatment plan to be formulated and then refined, and enough change to occur in a patient so that they can see and look forward to the future, it should not be denied.

How to Use this Book

There is tremendous personal power to be found in reemerging from an illness that has destabilized you and coming to terms with its impact on your life. This book is about what can and should be done to help individuals with neuropsychiatric brain disease begin and sustain this process. Chapters contain descriptions of Dr. Marotta's and The Lodge team's approach, interspersed with powerful accounts of personal experience written by former patients and Lodge alum parents that illustrate many of the diagnostic and treatment issues that The Lodge team feels need to be addressed for long-term stability to occur. At the end of each chapter, we have extracted key elements of The Lodge program that can be adapted by readers to support their own personal journey.

Neuropsychiatric brain disease is not one disease, and no two journeys will be exactly the same. But the underlying philosophy and approach to treatment presented in this book has application for the many faces of this illness, as does the intersectionality of themes such as relationship, collaboration, partnership, out-of-the-box thinking, the importance of medication, sobriety, persistence, and hope. This book does not give specific medical prescriptions or rules to be rigidly followed. Rather, it immerses the reader in the workings of The Lodge program because we believe that is the best way to share the important lessons that have been fundamental to its success. By the end of this book, we hope those who are struggling will feel less alone in their journey. We also hope you will understand that it is possible to be defined by much more than a diagnosis of neuropsychiatric brain disease, and to live a life filled with dignity and meaning.

"No one saw what we saw in the privacy of our home."

"The next 13 years were a roller coaster of 26 hospitalizations."

"The stigma of mental illness and the lack of guidance and support had left us feeling isolated and desperate."

"During my stay [at SHH] I relearned to love being alive."

"His "rights" trumped ours as his parents who were just trying to get him help."

"I did not think we would ever make it home safely."

"So, once again, we relied on the police."

"Then there was the allure of marijuana."

"Over the years he's been diagnosed by his doctor du jour with everything."

"A lack of insight about him having a mental illness made him challenging to treat and to parent."

"He also had side effects that troubled him."

"Getting the right combination of medications seemed hopeless. Feeling lost and without a solution I bottomed out."

"I pleaded with our insurance company to help...Their consulting psychiatrist...reminded me, "I'm not your friend.""

"When our son arrived at [SHH], Dr. Marotta...and his colleagues discovered a life threatening infection...

We believe this was just the beginning of how they saved his life."

"It was determined our son had an autoimmune disorder that was exacerbating his symptoms."

"Several psychiatrists in the past had given up on our son, calling his illness treatment-resistant.

Dr. Marotta would not give up on him. He searched for answers until he found them."

"We have always hoped he would have a purpose in his life as well as joy and to know he is loved...He is smiling again and so are we."

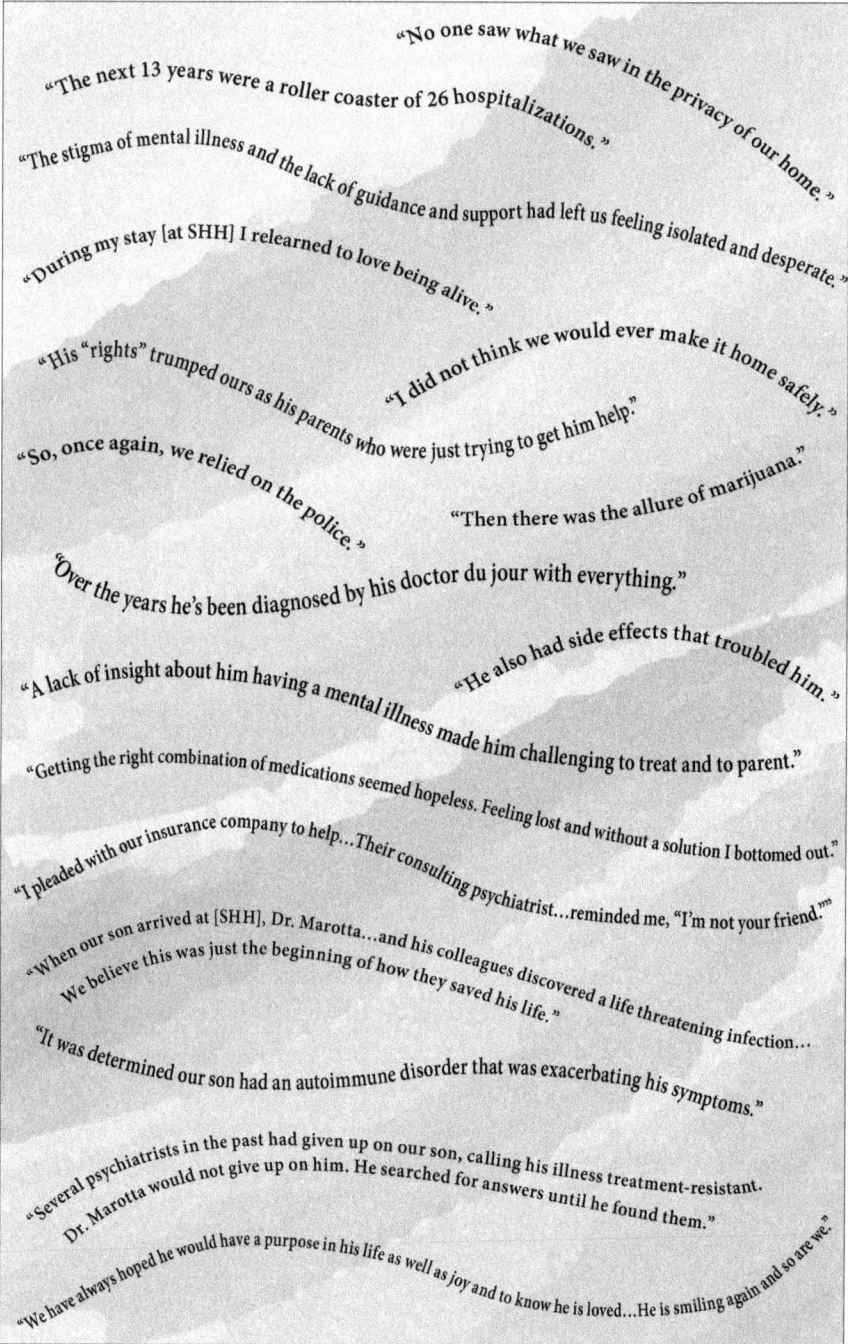

FIGURE 1: *Excerpts from personal stories*

Source: Silver Hill Hospital; background image source: "abstrack blue watercolor brush background Free Vector" from Vecteezy.com.

Chapter 1

THE VESSEL

"We may have all come on different ships,
but we're in the same boat now."

—*Martin Luther King, Jr.*

Navigating the journey through neuropsychiatric brain disease (NBD) is a complicated and complex task. It involves making sense of an array of symptoms; persuading a loved one to accept medications and, if possible, sobriety; helping them to develop a sense of agency; and ultimately reconnecting them to family and community. Finding a safe holding environment, a "vessel" in which all of this can take place, is the first building block to a positive outcome.

For some families, this boat, particularly in the early stages of illness, will be their own home. It will be a smaller vessel, harder to navigate and easier to damage. Thrust into the role of full-time caretakers and captain without much training, it is difficult and often overwhelming for family members to find a suitable crew. This often makes management of their loved one's illness fragmented due to no fault of their own.

The Lodge, part of the residential programs at Silver Hill Hospital, is a larger vessel and a model of fully integrated treatment. It provides a safe environment where care is highly customized for each patient's individual experience and peer modeling can occur. For families who can access The Lodge program, boarding this vessel is the first stage of a new journey for themselves and their loved ones. And for many, this vessel will be their home away from home for an extended period of time. How did this program evolve? It took time, experience, and a group of clinicians who refused to accept that the standard treatment of NBD was adequate to the needs of the NBD population of patients.

A Little History

Silver Hill Hospital (SHH) began its life as The Silver Hill Inn, established in 1931 by Dr. John A. P. Millet, who was looking for a site to which he could bring his private patients suffering from "nervous" disorders. "Guests" would reside there in the peaceful countryside for a period of time, seen by psychiatrists several times a week. They would engage in exercise and occupational therapy (arts and crafts or woodworking), have healthy, well-cooked, communal meals, make connections to other patients, and generally rest in the healing beauty of the private grounds. Over the decades, it became a fully incorporated hospital where patients could get treatment for a wider variety of psychiatric issues, with substance use disorders becoming a particular focus of treatment.

In earlier days, patients were not grouped according to diagnostic disorders. Over time, however, in response to the complexity of patient presentation and the growing medical understanding of diverse treatment modalities, staff teams were formed to focus on different types of issues. Dr. Marotta, a psychiatrist with a background in neuropsychology and brain physiology, had become the Service Chief of the Transitional Living Programs in 2008 and was impressed with the fact that patient symptoms often had to do with specific patterns of brain dysfunction. He and some of his colleagues resisted the accepted belief that schizophrenia had emerged from the disruption of a single area in the brain or that schizophrenia was even a single disease entity. Repeatedly, Dr. Marotta argued, "How can we have a treatment plan if we don't really know what the actual problem is?"

The current Lodge program (although called by a different name at that time) began to coalesce in its present form around 2010–2012, when the then-current president, Dr. Sigurd Ackerman, and his chief operating officer, Elizabeth Moore, suggested that a program might be developed for a few severely ill patients who did not fit into the profiles assigned to other treatment houses. These patients, who needed more help following their admission to the Acute Care Unit (ACU),* had nowhere to go that was appropriate to their needs. Patients enrolled in The Lodge program would learn to get up at a reasonable time, make their bed, to cook a meal, all while the staff thought carefully about their symptoms and their diagnosis.

Dr. Marotta had been sharing patients with staff all over the campus. A social worker, Wallace Stacy, LCSW, who had become interested in Dr. Marotta's belief that psychiatric disease should be approached as a constellation of symptoms rather than a single entity, transferred to The Lodge to work with him consistently, along with Joseph Silva, a residential counselor. Conversations with Dr. Marotta were always intriguing. He was a good listener and reveled in the exchange of ideas. Pocket watch swinging from a chain in his vest pocket, gray hair in a somewhat messy halo around his face, he talked patient diagnosis, neurobiology, art, and Greek history with anyone who wanted to listen. "You know, I was sitting beside Rocky on and off for a total of about thirteen years," said Mr. Stacey, now a former senior team member who continues a close relationship with the team and sees some of its discharged patients in his private practice. "He always pulled information about schizophrenia from old books, and he had the capacity to challenge what information you may have known about the illness without making you feel confronted. He is probably the wisest man I've ever spent time with. And he says, 'I don't know' more than any human I've ever met."

Dr. Marotta was earning a reputation for his specific approach to patient care. He was willing and interested in using multiple medications with patients, some off-label, to address their different symptoms. He often used clozapine, a powerful antipsychotic, which unfortunately few practitioners have the training or willingness to use. He called himself a "cowboy," monitoring his patients carefully but willing to take risks for potential long-term gains. For some staff, this way of working was too foreign but for others it was compelling. Increasingly, staff who shared patients with Dr. Marotta began to request that they continue to work with him on other cases. Slowly, gradually, the team that would consistently work together at The Lodge began to evolve. They knew they needed time

---

* The Acute Care Unit at Silver Hill Hospital is an eighteen-bed, locked inpatient hospital unit staffed twenty-four hours a day by physicians and nurses. Patients have single rooms, are supervised carefully, and reside there during the most acute phase of their illness.

with their patients in order to achieve breakthroughs. They were willing to fight with insurance companies and persuade families that extended stays in the program were critical for longer term gains. Slowly, the reputation of The Lodge as a place where remarkable outcomes could be achieved spread beyond the hospital campus, across time zones and overseas.

THE LODGE PROGRAM

Patients entering The Lodge have generally undergone multiple unsuccessful treatments or may have no clearly established diagnosis. Possible diagnoses can include schizophrenia spectrum disorders, affective spectrum disorders, and traumatic brain injury or other anatomical brain injuries resulting in the symptoms of NBD. Substance abuse is a frequent comorbidity. Coming on board to The Lodge most frequently involves a start in the ACU, where patients are evaluated and begin their treatment, often either in consultation with or under the direct care of a Lodge psychiatrist, who will be overseeing their care throughout their stay. Once a patient is deemed stable, with symptoms that are less externally disruptive to others in a therapeutic setting, they are taken over to the residential program at The Lodge. Work with patients at The Lodge is a multi-pronged approach, integrating medical, psychosocial, and occupational elements. Medical evaluation begins immediately with a rule out or rule in of underlying systemic physical issues, too often unexplored and undiagnosed when patients are sent to the hospital with unexplained or unremitting psychotic symptoms. If a physical issue is uncovered, addressing this issue becomes the first task of the team, and often requires collaboration with consultants and with family members, who need to follow through with getting the patient further testing.

The team sees each patient's illness as an individual puzzle that must be carefully solved, and at The Lodge, interventions are focused on particular symptoms and side effects rather than a diagnostic category. This is a very complex process and takes time. After a medication is begun, there must be time to assess its efficacy and associated side effects. Medications can be changed, dosages titrated up or down, and combinations carefully introduced. "Diagnoses are ideas," says Dr. Marotta. "We do not yet have precise pathophysiology. Therefore, we must accept that our formulations are provisional, and be willing to change course."

HOME AWAY FROM HOME

From the moment you enter The Lodge, it feels more like a home than a hospital or outpatient clinic. A white, two-story house perched at the end of a short path, its front lawn holds Adirondack chairs in a rainbow of colors, where residents can sit and socialize with each other or family members, groups can be held during beautiful weather, or lawn games played for relaxation and bonding. The foyer filled with coat racks, outdoor games, plants, and seasonal decor welcomes you into a light-filled common room which includes an electric fireplace, a television, piano, guitars, a kitchen for making snacks, meals, or hosting a cooking group, and a separate art area. Through the windows you can see the backyard, with its gazebo, patio furniture, and grill, a more sheltered place for quiet contemplation and connection. The residential counselors' office and a bathroom are located off the common room. Moving down two hallways are The Lodge's spacious bedrooms, which are each shared by two residents. Each is carpeted, with windows, two beds and bureaus, and two desks. At the end of one hallway downstairs is a smaller lounge area, where there is another television, games, and a washer and dryer. This room is also sometimes used by staff when they meet with the residents or their families. The medication administration room and nurse's office are located down the other hallway. Upstairs is another laundry room and offices, generally used by other hospital staff.

The Lodge can house up to fourteen residents, their stays mostly funded by their families. Many of the residents stay for six to twelve weeks and beyond. The Lodge is staffed around the clock. The team is comprised of three senior psychiatrists, two full-time social workers (plus interns), three full-time and many part-time residential counselors (and their interns), one full-time nurse, a couple of consulting psychologists who are able to do neuropsychological evaluations when requested, and often a medical student. Every team member describes their group as "an extended family." Dr. Marotta says, "I don't believe in hierarchies. If someone asked me about our team—which has a lot of people with advanced degrees on it—I call them 'our gang.' It's like we're in this together." One team member, when asked what it is like to work at The Lodge, replied, "At The Lodge, there is no big I, little you."

The Importance of a Calm Environment

The Lodge is not a locked residence, and to live there, patients must be assessed as not dangerous to themselves or others. But many of the residents come to The Lodge with active hallucinations and delusions still strongly in place. Their hold on reality is compromised, and unpredictable environments with the potential for high emotional input are stressful. At The Lodge, the staff monitor and adjust physical and emotional distance based on patients' needs rather than prescribed requirements. They create a calm, safe environment where social behavior is encouraged but not pushed. "I try to make [The Lodge] a very calm environment," says Curtina Alexander, LPCA, the senior Residential Counselor (RC). "Nobody can function in dysfunction, psychotic or not. So, I feel like the atmosphere, your surroundings, play a very big role in that. I tell people, when you happen to look good, you feel better. So, when you're in a safe, comfortable environment, you start to feel safe."

Getting residents to take medication is also considered a first priority, because the staff knows that the development of trust in the treatment process is dependent on reducing positive symptoms (again, things like hallucinations, delusions, and distortions in thinking) and increasing rational awareness. Particularly when you are on a medication like clozapine that requires repeated blood work and regulation of side effects, if you do not trust your doctors and are not convinced of the drug's efficacy, there is little incentive to continue to take it. This is a very complex interaction. Patients are struggling to maintain autonomy and agency. When they arrive, they are placed in a situation where they must surrender to the judgment of others, despite their own perceptions. "It is a difficult dance," says Dr. Marotta. "It cannot be accomplished by commanding a patient to do what you say." If a patient is discharged before this trust can develop and does not get this support from somewhere else, the probability that severe symptoms will reappear over time is high.

The Community

The Lodge is a place where patient goals are dynamic, not static. Feedback from anyone, regardless of role, is always welcomed, and families are given full access to each member of The Lodge team. The community is an extended one, reaching out to include AA sponsors, staff at residential or step-down housing,* consultants, or anyone else who interacts with the patients, including housekeeping, who often give some of the most useful information. To fit with the team, you must be patient and kind, a good listener who respects feedback from all sources, especially the patients themselves.

For example, two alums of The Lodge noted that taking oxytocin before work meetings at their jobs allowed them to overcome their social anxiety and speak with ease. This idea prompted Dr. Marotta to change oxytocin dosing schedules in the program, where many members participate in groups and now feel better able to speak because they take their oxytocin beforehand. "An essential feature of doing what you do," says Dr. Marotta, "is that you are always trying to understand more. In the service of that, you're always reading, you're always comparing, you're always engaging with other people who might have a different perspective, a different knowledge than you do. There is always a constant search to understand."

None of this could occur, however, without the time and space needed to work. Safety is also always an issue, given the severity of the diseases being treated and the degree of impairment they cause. The calm, safe environment provided by an extended stay as part of The Lodge "family" is considered foundational to the success of this program. The team protects this calm environment at all costs.

THE CENTER FOR THE TREATMENT AND STUDY OF NEUROPSYCHIATRIC DISORDERS

The work taking place at The Lodge has generated enormous excitement and raised important questions that need to be studied. What are the elements that are most transformative in this multifaceted experience? Can it be replicated without an extended stay hospital structure? How can The Lodge team's process best be shared and taught? These and other questions are foundational to the creation of The Center for the Treatment and Study of Neuropsychiatric Disorders at Silver Hill Hospital. Directed by Dr. Marotta, its mission is to take what has been learned from The Lodge team's experience and expand it outward. Currently, there are two

---

* Residential or step-down communities are post-hospital residences that provide varying degrees of structure and supervision after someone has been discharged from an inpatient hospitalization. They are described in greater detail in Chapter Eight: Safe Harbors.

research collaborations that are underway, along with continued conference presentations, articles and teaching Rounds. The Center is funded by
grateful families, who generously want others to benefit from the expertise
that has brought them hope where previously there was little.

Plans are also underway to bring the model of treatment outlined in
this book to the Bridgeport Rescue Mission, to help vulnerable members
of a complex, inner-city population through the operation of a free community health-care clinic, Sage Healthcare. This novel program provides
for local university faculty and students in various health-care disciplines
to identify clients with the diagnosis of schizophrenia, and to implement
a detailed clozapine treatment protocol, manage side effects, adjunctive
medications, and evaluate outcomes through the use of psychosis rating
scales. Group therapy, family engagement, as well as the supportive structure of Bridgeport Rescue Mission itself, are being designed to emulate
The Lodge program. Experienced SHH clinicians will play a major role
in the development and support of this program. The goal is to replicate
in the community a residential setting through which patients can be followed daily, treated primarily with clozapine, and returned to long-term
stability and a meaningful life. See the Appendix for more detailed information about projects occurring at the Center.

Putting It All Together

To stick with our metaphor, in the midst of a storm, not all vessels
are equally seaworthy. Some programs, like leaky boats, will be inadequate to the needs of their passengers, capsizing quickly and lacking
suitable lifeboats to row their passengers to shore. We think The
Lodge program is a model of the type of vessel needed to weather the
acute phase of NBD, made particularly seaworthy by the efforts of
its captain and its crew, who maintain the integrity of the structure.
What makes this vessel particularly sturdy? It is not the fact that it is
cosmetically impressive, but rather that it is built in such a way that
the passengers feel safe, protected, and spend enough time on board
to develop their equilibrium. The staff of The Lodge program work
hard to create a particular type of environment for their patients.
Here are the key elements that help to make a program's environment
more successful.

KEY IDEAS FOR CHAPTER ONE: THE VESSEL

- Programs for individuals with NBD should provide a calm, safe environment where social behavior is encouraged but not pushed.

- The approach of the program should integrate medical, psychosocial, and occupational elements.

- Clinicians who work within a program need to share frequent feedback; feedback from all staff, including from nonclinical members of the team and the patients themselves, is welcomed.

- A program should show flexibility of response to the needs of a patient rather than adherence to rigid ideological rules.

- Programs should extend their community to include partnerships with organizations like AA, and residential and step-down communities.

"Silver Hill Hospital Was not Our First Rodeo"

—A Parent's Story

In early summer of 2020, my son was taken by hospital-arranged transport from an involuntary stay at a behavioral health and substance use disorder treatment hospital in NJ to a voluntary admission in CT at Silver Hill Hospital's Transitional Living Program at The Lodge. He was 23 years old, out of control at home with substance use, suicidal ideations, mania, and in the midst of his third psychotic break, where the new current delusion was that he had been molested by his mother.

Silver Hill Hospital was not our first rodeo. There were fourteen years preceding the Silver Hill Hospital admission where my son suffered first in silence and later in vocal anguish, but always to the puzzlement of his parents, friends, teachers, and medical providers. Diagnoses that were posited piled up: ADHD, auditory processing disorder, sensory integration disorder, dysthymic disorder, generalized anxiety disorder, social anxiety disorder, major depression disorder, borderline personality, cannabis misuse disorder, drug-induced psychosis, mixed episode bipolar with psychotic features, and schizoaffective disorder. In the preceding five years, there were four hospitalizations, a three-month stay in a wilderness therapy program in a Western state, a six-month long stay in a sober living facility in another, and two outpatient treatments through an East Coast program for psychotic illness. All through the years, my son had a deep distrust of and lack of connection with most treatment providers and medications. As his mother, I often felt frustrated, misunderstood, and degraded within the realm of the educational and mental health systems. Paradoxically, much of my exasperation, however, was ultimately directed toward my son.

In order to get my adult son to Silver Hill Hospital, it required my husband and I to have unconditional love, yet the courage to face some stark truths. Our previous experiences with hospitalizations for mental illness were pretty dismal. Naïve to the system, at first, I thought hospitals were the place you went to get the answers about illness and recover one's mental health. The experience to date had been much different. The previous hospitals' focus appeared to be on keeping our son safe, calm, and not a disruption to other patients, and [patients] medically stabilized where they were deemed not a danger to themselves or others, therefore "ready for discharge." What this usually meant was a steady stream of a benzo-

Continued ➤

diazepine so our son would be cooperative, then perhaps heavy doses of a mood stabilizer, and finally pick an antipsychotic and hope that it will work out in the long run. Three to fourteen days later, he would be discharged with a paper prescription for medicine and instructions to follow up on his own accord with the next treatment provider or outpatient program. Our son was certainly never healed upon discharge; in retrospect, not even "well." As parents of a young adult, we were often left out of the discharge process yet expected to take care of him after with no guidance on long-term recovery.

The previous discharges were downright scary. My son made it home from a discharge in Colorado and within one day he went without his medication and was back in a mixed-manic state, and with a "friend" who thought a "welcome home" with cocaine was in order. Back on the medications prescribed, he slept twelve to fourteen hours each day, could not drive, could not concentrate, had no pleasure in movies, television, or games, and had an inner restlessness, with leg shaking and constant thirst.

At the First Episode Psychosis Center, the outpatient program was consumer-centered, meaning that my son had control over the amount, duration, and scope of his treatment. Freshly out of the hospital, he met once a week with a recovery coach, who was still in pursuit of a master's degree, and once a month with their psychiatric mental health nurse practitioner, who was in charge of medication. The program did not have evening hours and was closed on the weekends. The program's goal to change the trajectory of the illness through timely treatment so that the consumer can continue to pursue their occupational, educational, and social goals was a positive one. In practice, however, this takes a lot more care, consideration, and skill [on the part] of [the] professionals to accomplish. Pursuing his desires, my son was off medication in three months and employed full-time in a job, with hours that prevented him from continuing in the program. A few months later, with a letter in hand from the program stating he could go back to pursue his studies at his out-of-state university, he was readmitted to school that fall. Seven weeks later, he was hospitalized with a second break.

In the following spring, while living at home now and attending the local community college, our son was hospitalized with his third break. This time, we held firm with the hospital that there could be no unsafe discharge to our home. The hospital social worker presented a 28-day substance recovery program to our son. We recognized, however, that our son

Continued ➤

was still delusional, needed lifesaving treatment, and a relationship with his parents in his life was crucial. After reading Dr. Marotta's online bio, where he says, "we never give up here," we knew, as parents, we were in line with that thinking. We presented Silver Hill Hospital, instead, as our choice for long-term residential treatment, and luckily the hospital's doctor recognized this as the opportunity of a lifetime.

Immediately Silver Hill Hospital was different. Whereas the previous hospital discharged our son as being stable, it was immediately recognized by Silver Hill staff that our son was still in mania and psychosis, and he was transferred up to the Main building. The medication initiated at Main pulled him out of it but had some terrible physical side effects.

The transfer to Dr. Marotta's care at The Lodge was seamless. Apparently, the team was keeping an eye on him and assessing his readiness. I remember Rocky explaining to us that our son was like a boxer who needed a lot of time in a healing environment to rest his brain now. Rocky was confident in a non-arrogant way. He was very reassuring that there was a lot of hope that with time, the right medication, and staying away from substances, that the brain could reset. I had amassed a mountain of collateral information to supply the team with, but to my surprise the team of Rocky and Wallace [Stacey] did not seem puzzled by it or even that interested in it. It was the present symptoms that they focused on and not a particular diagnosis. Apparently, they recognized a "thought disorder" when they saw it, something I had never even heard of before.

It was explained to us that Rocky had a lot of experience and success with using clozapine, and it should have less physical side effects than the current medication he was on; but it came with a different set of challenges that required a high degree of expertise, time, and patience to find the right dosage. It was my son, however, who made the decision. I heard that Rocky was able to find a connection with my son regarding his desire to feel "smart again," which was something of which my son took pride. According to Wallace, his social worker, my son ultimately decided to go for it after posing the question in the group therapy with his young adult peers in the house, "Should I try clozapine?"

Changing to clozapine permanently got rid of my son's extrapyramidal side effects from the other medication. It also allowed him to drop the mood stabilizer. In the beginning, he was very tired, slept a lot, and presented in his typical monosyllabic way with us. Rocky let us know that sleep was good for his brain and that the difference with clozapine is that it

Continued ➤

has protective qualities for brain cells, and he has seen continuing improvement in patients up to a year later.

The combined approach of Rocky's optimism and Wallace's realism worked symbiotically. Initially feeling pressure that time was slipping away from our son's ability to start his life at 23 years old, the team at Silver Hill provided us the space to understand that it was important to be patient and that the outcome was not predetermined. Family support, continuity of care, medication compliance, and continued healing of the brain from substances and toxic environments was paramount. They did not discount or elevate my son's goal to go to college. If it happened, it would happen when his brain was ready.

They were also patient with our own anxieties and provided the answers we needed:

Q: How will he be able to do school without ADHD medication?

A: *He never had ADHD.*

Q: How will it work to need weekly blood testing?

A: *He will get used to it.*

Q: Doesn't my son owe me an apology for his molestation delusion?

A: *Why? He was sick. Would you expect an apology from a cancer survivor?*

Q: Do we have to explore his delusions to recover?

A: *Only if your son brings it up. Otherwise let it go.*

Q: Does our son need cognitive remediation?

A: *Let's do a comprehensive psychological evaluation after being on clozapine.*

Q: What is the cause of psychotic illness?

A: *There is an underlying genetic vulnerability that physical and psychological stressors can bring out.*

Q: How important is it to stay away from marijuana and stimulant medication when you have a psychotic illness?

A: *It's like playing with fire.*

After leaving The Lodge, my son transitioned to a small-group residence for men with mental health disorders, where he was very fortunate to continue on with Rocky and Wallace as the treatment team. The group

Continued ➤

residence's advisors had a lot of experience in dealing with young men starting clozapine. They knew what to expect out of our son and were very encouraging. Rocky augmented the clozapine regimen with oxytocin in order to enhance the overall healing process. The psychological assessment was completed and found no cognitive deficits. In fact, our son's IQ went up twenty points from the one completed a few years before. Later, Wallace recommended a wonderful educational coach to get our son back slowly into classes.

Rocky's ability to connect with my son is nothing short of amazing. My perspective is that his confidence, caring, effectiveness of treatment, and approachability have engendered my son's trust. I don't know the context, but my son mentioned that Rocky once said to him, "Hey, I stick my neck out for you," and apparently that created quite an impression. Ultimately, I really appreciate that Rocky's approach is to treat the whole person. He addresses my son's concerns from weight loss to wheezing to social anxiety with girls.

Today is the three-year anniversary of my son meeting Dr. Marotta and the treatment team at Silver Hill and the beginning of his clozapine medication. While the coveted first girlfriend experience has eluded him and contributes to moments of high anxiety, he reaches out directly to Rocky or another trusted person and now recovers more quickly from these states. His overall recovery has been impressive. We don't focus on the "diagnosis," and recently my son told me he thinks he's bipolar but that "Rocky doesn't really answer him about 'what he has' but that he currently knows he has some sort of anxiety disorder." My son puts me on the spot about what I think he has, and I say, "My understanding is it's a spectrum disorder: bipolar, schizoaffective, schizophrenia." With this response, my son brightly asks me if I know what "spectrum" means and enthusiastically explains that it means it has a wide range so that it's very individualized to the person!

This summer, he is a full-time paid intern at an engineering firm and enjoys living, for the first time in three years, back with his parents. In the fall, he will be 26 years old and entering his final year toward a civil engineering degree from a university where he takes pride that he was selected into the National Engineering Honors Society.

In college, my son lives in a house with students who he now calls "friends" and refers to himself humorously as being "old as f--k." He says that while he would love Rocky to be at his graduation, he "knows Rocky is a really busy guy!" And when questioned about the challenges of obtaining and taking his clozapine, his response is "I have to do what I have to do."

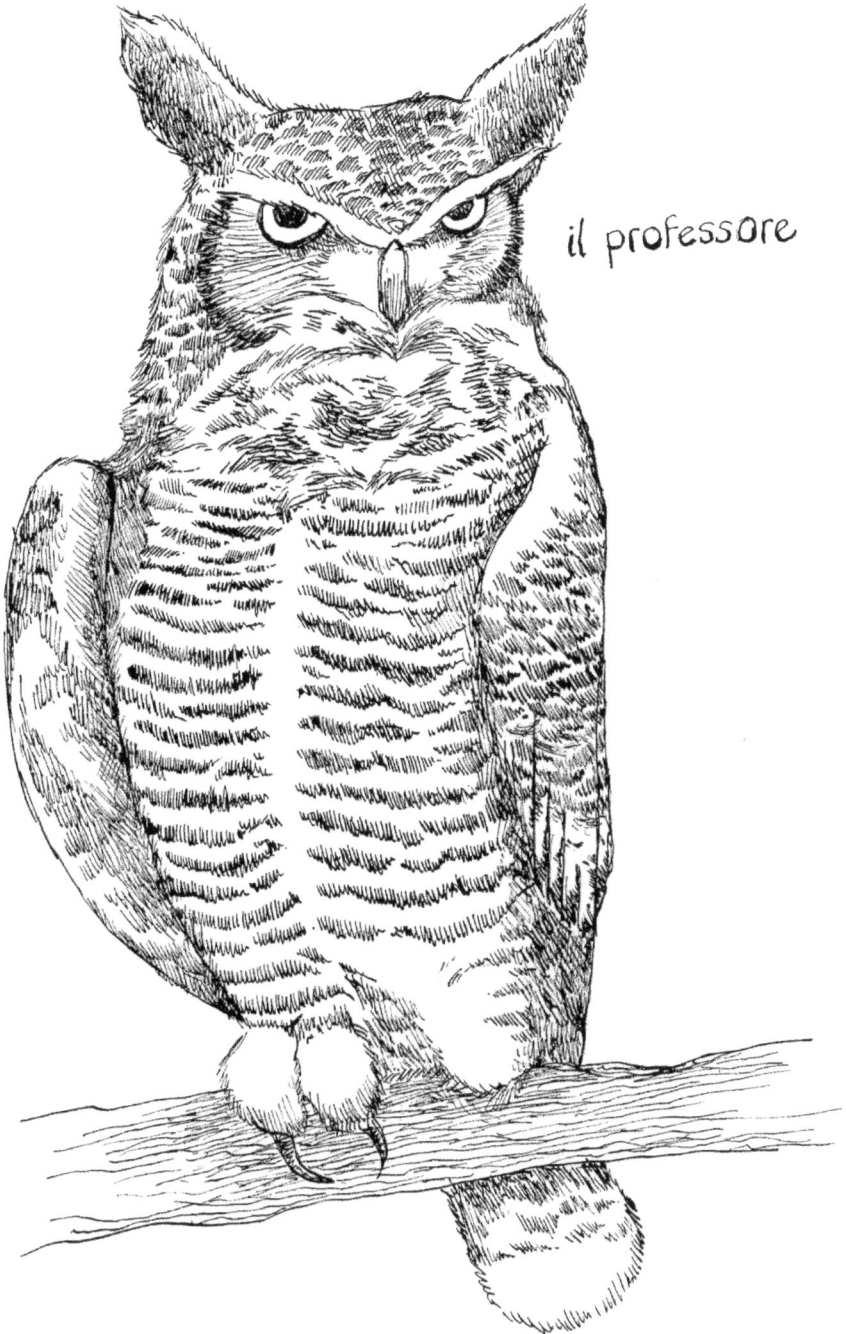

il professore

FIGURE 2: *The Owl drawing*

Source: Gift to Rocky from the artist; used with permission of the artist.

Chapter 2

THE CAPTAIN

"A Toast: to Continuing the Work!"

—*Dr. Rocco Marotta*

It is a dark and stormy night.... Well, a dark and stormy day. The rain is torrential. Flood alerts abound. "Is it still on?" Texts from Lodge staff members to Dr. Marotta about the party he is hosting fly back and forth, interspersed with "Can I bring my mother who is visiting?" and "Would it be OK to bring my children?"

"Of course, the party is still on, and family is more than welcome," he texts back. During his childhood, extended family and friends often descended, unannounced, for Sunday visits to his Italian-American family's home in Queens. That kind of easy welcome reflects the important value of relationship that he has inherited. In his Connecticut home, on the day of the party, the tables have been rearranged from outside to in, garage doors have been opened for easier access to the house from the driveway, and candles have been lit to assuage the ominous darkness and sheets of rain. It is a day that requires adaptive thinking, acceptance of the present moment, and a positive reframe. But will the staff really come? It's hideous outside, a much better day to stay at home and curl up with a book, a movie, or a video game.

First one person, then a few more begin to trickle in. As time goes on, almost the entire staff, even some who have left the program for other jobs and have driven distances to come, brave the elements and fill the house with their laughter and earnest conversation. Who are these people and why did they venture out when weather forecasters were telling people to stay at home? Most importantly, what relevance does this party have to the issue of neuropsychiatric brain disease and its successful treatment?

There are some themes in this book which you will hear about repeatedly, because from all accounts they stand out as essential components in a successful treatment journey. Perhaps the most important is the ineffable element of enduring relationships, both between staff and patients and among team members themselves whose sense of connection to each other helps to create a safe and positive environment for the patients. Riding through sheets of rain on your day off requires more than enjoyment of each other's company. It requires the loyalty of steadfast connection and a belief that you are valued. Dr. Marotta—"Rocky," "Doc Roc"—is a father figure to some, to others a spiritual advisor, and to all a mentor.

Staff stand around the kitchen island, contemplating the cake that has a banner reading "A Toast: to Continuing the Work!" and listening to the man that drew most of them to The Lodge program. "How do we describe what we do? The words don't matter," Rocky says. "What matters is that our actions show that we care for each other, that we support one another, that we support our patients and their families no matter what." He is true to his words. Despite the demanding, often frustrating, and sometimes heartbreaking work that they do, they know he always has their back. And patients and families agree: Rocky will be there no matter what, encouraging, cajoling, educating, comforting, in it for the long haul. For many, this is the magic glue that holds their recovery together, whether they are moving forward, sometimes backward, or paddling to stay in place.

Who is this man who navigates the ship, even in stormy weather? We will introduce you to the proverbial captain of this ship in a moment, but first a cautionary note. There are many ways to be an effective clinician, and part of the successful functioning of The Lodge team is that each team member is free to work in their own personal style with patients. Rocky talks about his team with reverence and enormous respect, not because they are his clones, but precisely because each of them is different from him and brings their own clinical sensitivity and skill to the table. Conversely, it is Rocky's unique clinical style that every member of the team says has inspired them to embrace their own new approach to the work. This chapter aims to give you a peephole into Rocky's personal style, and a greater understanding of the man whose vision has been foundational to the development of The Lodge program. We remind you, however, that the success of this program stems not from one individual's work but from the collaborative experience of many.

ROCKY

"The good physician treats the disease; the great physician treats the patient who has the disease."

—*Attributed to Sir William Osler, MD*

Rocco Marotta, MD, PhD, is just as likely to be called "Doc Roc" as he is "Dr. Marotta." In fact, he calls himself "Rocky," and his personal email reads "olddocroc." At 75 years of age, growing up in the working-class neighborhoods of New York City, he is equally at home talking to a patient about their home-town parish as he is mentoring younger colleagues or giving Grand Rounds on a complex clinical or psychopharmacological issue. Rocky has dedicated his life to helping those in need but believes healing takes many forms and is never rigid.

Most staff on the Silver Hill Hospital campus know Rocky personally, but even if they don't, they could pick him out of a lineup with his iconic three-piece suit, clogs or boots with one pant leg tucked inside and the other flowing free. In some ways his look sums up a lot about him—his nod to the "traditional," but his idiosyncratic take on things, his charming eccentricity, his willingness to buck the norm. Rocky looks more like an absent-minded professor than a stereotypical hospital doctor. His office is messy, filled with files and piles of paperwork. There is artwork on the walls and cards, many of them owls, pinned to a corkboard. Most importantly, patients and staff know that underneath that eclectic style is an ability to absorb and integrate information that can be lifesaving.

Rocky laughs easily with patients and colleagues because he isn't afraid to be himself. He can be firm, gentle, humorous, serious, elated, irritated, but always understanding, real and present. Administrators find him frustrating (he is suspicious of algorithms and is not technologically savvy), colleagues find him helpful (his ability to solve resistant medical dilemmas is well known), families find him responsive (he almost always picks up phone calls, no matter the time of day or night), patients find him a rescuer (he is considered the doctor who never gives up). This is, of course, a simplified version of the truth. Rocco Marotta, MD, PhD, is a unique figure, someone who defies simple description, whose complexity is founded on a lifetime of wildly diverse experiences.

To understand Rocky and his development of The Lodge and The Lodge's team, it is helpful to understand a bit about his personal history. The son of second-generation, working-class Italian-American parents, Rocky's childhood was filled with copious food and enthusiastic discussion around a table, the model of hard work and stoicism, family members who all served as soldiers, an unconditionally loving mother, and a Catholic worldview, overseen by priestly fathers and mother nuns. Rocky has always had a curious mind and was the first of his family to go to college. He has always been a reader and a seeker of knowledge. But his role models are from early life: "my father, my grandfather ... who told me life is filled with dangers, but you have to engage ... to act brave." Fascinated by the brain and behavior, Rocky became a psychologist before he became a physician, eventually researching recovery from brain trauma with the use of psychopharmacological medications long before he knew he would become a psychiatrist. He went to medical school in his thirties, already a scholar of neuroanatomy and brain physiology. Now, in his seventies, his belief in the Hippocratic Oath continues to be unwavering. When he works with a patient, his mission is to heal and protect. "You have to be a physician first," he says. "You have to care for the patient in every way possible. Our vocation is to do more than categorize, fill out forms, and write scripts. As my Uncle Arty, who was a marine, would say, 'It is our job to not leave the wounded behind.'"

CORE APPROACH

It is difficult to capture the nature of Rocky's working process because it changes to fit the needs of each individual patient. When asked to describe how he evaluates a patient, Rocky says, "My mind works in stories; it doesn't work in terms of lists." However, at the core is the general principle that what is to be treated is a constellation of symptoms, not a diagnosis. "I don't believe in statistical cutoffs. I believe in individuals. We don't think of one drug as being the answer. Thirty-five years ago, it was a big thing to pay attention to dual diagnoses. Now it is quadruple diagnoses."

Rocky is always looking for reasons treatment might have failed, and failure to achieve results is seen not as a defeat but as a source of information, a waypoint on the path to success. What could have been missed? What could be tried that is different? "Sometimes treating professionals are so sure of a diagnosis that they don't go back to the beginning and ask, What are the other possibilities that might so disrupt someone's brain that they would behave in a certain way that looks schizophrenic or severely bipolar or looks like a personality disorder? Could it really be epilepsy? Could it really be an autoimmune disease? Could it really be a genetic malformation or a tumor? Could it be a horrible trauma that has not been articulated? And so, I am always perplexed, amused, amazed how often certain things aren't done."

Rocky is well known for his out-of-the-box thinking—his "mental resilience," as one colleague put it—and for battling a reimbursement system that pulls for quick diagnoses and fewer questions asked. Getting necessary imaging and bringing in appropriate consultations takes enormous time, energy, and experience. It is not unusual for him to order EEGs (e.g., certain types of epilepsy can cause psychosis and EEGs show epilepsy), PET scans, MRIs of the brain (e.g., to check for certain kinds of subtle dementias), antinuclear antibody tests (e.g., an ANA test may reveal autoimmune disease, which may be a critical factor), and any other blood tests that look at blood chemistry (infections can impair cognition). Rocky is curious about discrepancies, for example, strong past educational functioning in a person who now shows no ability to think abstractly. Importantly, he is not afraid to bring a different perspective to a discussion. Thinking aloud he says:

> Your mind has to say, *Could it be this, this, and this, or none of these, or a mix of them? And is there a test for that?*" And (maybe) your guesses were wrong. Now what's left? What could it be? And you're constantly saying—at least I'm constantly saying to myself—*What's really going on?* And the failures become great puzzles, and that ties into the whole thing of not giving up. Not letting yourself give up, being hopeful, and then helping the patient and the family not to give up either.

This model of out-of-the-box thinking has had a definite impact on the team, where the sharing of ideas and dialogue are encouraged. "Rocky has taught me to think differently," said Jackie Ordoñez, LCSW, a senior team member, who says her professional creativity has blossomed working at The Lodge. In this program there is room for persuasive argument and debate. There is also a willingness to reevaluate in the face of failure and to understand that patience is required when you are taking new paths toward change.

FINDING A WAY IN

During a family meeting not so long ago, Rocky was asking a patient's father about his own history. The father mentioned he went to one of the military academies. Rocky asked him, "What class?" And when it turned out he graduated class of 1970, Rocky exclaimed, "That was my class!" and told him the story of how he desperately wanted to go to West Point and why he didn't get there. "And at this point," said Rocky, "we were friends for life."

Rocky seeks clarity at the very start of treatment about the problem the patient or family wants him to solve. Expectations and hopes vary from family to family. "I was raised by marines," he often says in initial interviews, "I need a mission. I want orders." Goals of treatment can always evolve, but an initial plan of action needs to be clear and shared by the doctor, team, patient, and their family. The search for points of commonality is then the first step toward building a relationship with a patient and their family. For this he pulls from every aspect of his own life experience—his reading and fascination with diverse subjects, his childhood, and his current family life. While he doesn't tell families everything, Rocky shares vignettes of his life generously, and empathizes with their struggle. "I say to them, 'I'm an old guy and what I've noticed over the years. . . .' And [this makes us] kind of equals in the struggle. It is important to overcome the sense of fear and isolation that fuels the underlying paranoia of these illnesses. You have to be able to touch the underlying sense of shared humanity." It is a gentle approach, one that has made Rocky particularly skilled at connecting with withdrawn and anxious people. For example, the young man who wouldn't speak to anyone until Rocky talked to him about the Yankees.

"He was born in the Bronx," relates Rocky, "and I said, 'God, you're just a few blocks from the stadium, what do you think of blah, blah, blah?' That opened it up. In talking about baseball you could do a mental status exam, and you could do just about anything you need[ed] to. You have to find a hook. [Communicate] that you're [both] human beings, that you share something."

With one patient it might be baseball, another it might be cooking, a third it might be poetry or philosophy, but in every conversation, he is always assessing—is someone chatting or quiet? Are they overly literal or tangential? Related or withdrawn? A colleague described it well:

> Rocky fully holds people in his presence, and as much as he asks them about their lives, he also opens up about his. Long-term patients know all about how his mother lived with his sister, and about his grandchildren, his dog, and all sorts of pieces of his life. It is a real connection that is so absent in most doctor-patient relationships. Rocky makes himself vulnerable as he talks of loss in his own life and always inserts lightness as he refers to his grandchildren. Of course, in between conversations about life he is able to comment about the patient's well-being, current symptoms and concerns, along with peppering in his clinical opinions.
>
> A patient comes to a session, and by the end of the half-hour, Rocky has masterfully led them to agree to a medication change, or to securing an appointment with their specialist, or to stay the course of treatment. At another moment, a past patient visits and before long, Rocky is talking about the drug epidemic, cultural trends in alcoholism, and then this leads to talk about a trip this patient took, and Rocky then discussing the early explorers, Columbus, the discovery of the Strait of Magellan and more.
>
> This is just forty-five minutes in Rocky's day, filled with continuous phone calls either to hospital staff, consultants, patients and their families, Rounds, and numerous visitors popping in to touch base or seeking advice, as he continues to work with his assistant on tomorrow's presentation and research.

Being "Sneaky," or the Indirect Approach

When asked to talk about his process with patients, Rocky uses the word "sneaky" a surprising number of times. For someone who believes in being direct with families and who is often described by others as "authentic" in his work with patients, it is an interesting turn of phrase and begs elaboration. Rocky calls his approach "sneaky" because he is always looking to gain or give information without his patients feeling interrogated or "pressed to confess."

Patients at The Lodge often enter SHH hospital in a withdrawn, disorganized, or defensively mute state. They can be resistant to admitting they hear voices or are experiencing bizarre delusions. They are often isolated inside their head and ashamed of feeling so different. These things are roadblocks to getting necessary information. Rocky's Old Doc Roc persona is not authoritarian or dictatorial. "I don't say, 'I'm the doctor, you have to take your medicine.' I'll say things like, 'I think that you are hearing voices, and the voices are telling you to say, "No, I don't have voices!"'' I'm a strange, crazy, old guy. What I've noticed is that the voices are a parasite. They don't want you to get better." As the captain of the ship on which they are now sailing, he will always be honest about the storms that they are facing. But Rocky's message is clear. He is in the boat with his passengers and has no plans to leave them on the ship alone.

BEING PERPLEXED

Sometimes being "perplexed" is a better way to get a patient to elaborate than asking outright. Watching patients interacting in the dining room, listening to what residents are saying as he sits in the nursing station, or watching them interact with the little dog he sometimes brings to work, are also often better ways to gather information than asking checklist questions. That is why you can often find Rocky and members of the team just hanging with the residents. And when he can use humor, Rocky teases and jokes and is playful, his giggle often echoing down the hallway. "You've got to pull yourself together, Agent G," he tells one agitated patient who he has been teasing about being a spy. "What kind of an agent are you? You have to be calm and focused . . . you're gonna blow this whole thing!" And G laughs and says, "Ah, okay."

Rocky is, by his own report, often having a "grand time" with his patients, but he is always assessing the best way to help them move forward. Sometimes it means helping them to understand that it is okay not to be conventional. Sometimes that means helping them understand what more normal behavior looks like. "Being perplexed is a way of acknowledging that you do not have all the answers, and we often don't," Rocky says. "That doesn't mean that we can't try to understand and to help."

He also adds that it is important to recognize that the vast majority of patients do not want to be in the hospital. They have lost control of their lives; they want to be free, to have autonomy, to be like everyone else. Sometimes he coaches them on how to behave normally.

> I'll say, "I know you really want to get out of the hospital, so this is how we have to fool the staff." I just did that with X last week. I said, "X, you've been in so long, you really got to get out, I know you really want to. I know you're better, but you have to start acting better. You know when your therapist comes to see you, you can't say nothing! You have to go to groups and take part. You can't just meditate in the corner." Later, one of the social workers came to see me, and she said, "Dr. So-and-so called to say they had the most amazing session. [X] told her all kinds of things. Dr. So-and-so asked, 'Did you change his medicine?' I said, 'No, no, Dr. Marotta just told him, if he wanted to get discharged, he had to start acting normal.'"

Encouraging Rehearsal of Normal Behavior; Active Cheerleading

In fact, rehearsal of normal behavior is an important part of the process of reintegration into the wider community, and the team fully supports involvement in communities like AA, where patients can make friends and practice being with others. When a patient is ready to try school or a job, Rocky often assumes the role of life coach, cheerleader, and even tutor. Conversations like this often involve an element of cognitive remediation, helping them to think through and think about how they can approach complex or difficult tasks. He talks to them about choices, sometimes giving them cautionary tales from his own life. He helps them to think through writing assignments for classes, gives them concrete advice about how to handle studying, and tells them, "I didn't finish medical school until I was 40! It's never too late." When patients leave The Lodge, Rocky actively calls those who don't call him, because passivity is a hallmark of this spectrum of disorders and is not seen as resistance. "Very often they don't reach out to me," says Rocky. "I reach out to them ... but a lot of them say, 'I really appreciate that you hunt me down. That [you check to see] that I'm ok.'"

The Importance of Connection

Connection can take many forms but is fundamental to a successful outcome. Therapy is not a conventional forty-five-minute therapy hour. It can be a weekly fifteen-minute check-in to evaluate if everything is going well or a long conversation about life and a school paper. When his patients are discharged from the hospital, Rocky is famous for making "spur-of-the-moment" telephone calls just to touch base. Patients may have very little or a lot to say, but that doesn't worry him. It allows him to get a sense from their voice as to how things are going and whether or not he needs to take any further action. Most importantly, it sends the message that he is thinking about them and is available if they need him, just as his frequent use of the word "we" when talking about how things are going (e.g., "How are we doing?") reflects a partnership rather than a hierarchical relationship. And while some patients call at inappropriate hours, Rocky accepts this with good humor. On the one hand, it may be part of a difficulty picking up on social cues, often part of NBD. On the other, it may reflect a family dynamic that has been transferred to their relationship. In either case, he understands that his patients' sense of connection is part of the glue that holds their lives together. It is well worth occasional lapses in boundaries.

Involving Patients in Their Own Treatment

In every way possible, Rocky encourages his patients to be active participants in their own treatment. Regaining a sense of agency and taking responsibility is central to his patients' success. It is also critical that they don't feel abandoned. "Getting them to help us help them gives them power," he says, "and that gives them pride in the process."

Sometimes he will say, "Your job is to keep track of what's wrong. Because I'm the kind of foolish person who will miss it." Other times he reminds them, "You know I am a cheerleader, and since I am a cheerleader, I am always emphasizing what's good, [and] you have to be very careful that I know if anything is wrong."

And how does he think they see him? "I'm like the grandfather they're protective of in some fashion. And, once [our relationship] goes on over months, I think they're staying on track for my sake, to keep me going. They're trying to get better, but it's a balancing game. And that's why

[I do] these conversations. I call them [and say], 'This is a pep talk and you have to do this and this and this.' They and their families have suffered so much. The kids have to learn to take risks again." For Lodge patients this is often complicated. They are often four to eight years or more behind their peers in the pursuit of school and work. This makes rejoining the "conventional" world particularly challenging.

THE TEACHER WHO SEEKS TO BE TAUGHT

Dr. Marotta's office is filled with cards of appreciation and gratitude from patients and their families. His perseverance and guidance have gotten so many through rough travels. But when asked to speak about his patient experiences, he is more apt to talk about what they have taught him than what he has done for them. Experience with one patient has highlighted how there is always more history to learn, despite hours of conversation. Another has taught him "about the virtuous cycle of getting better, that by taking small risks and succeeding, it allows one to move forward and not feel defeated." Another has taught him that transference* can be just as powerful in brain illnesses as it is in traditionally "neurotic" dysfunction. And yet others have taught him to be subtle when family is intrusive, or to be more assertive when rehearsal of interpersonal connection is important. In every case, Dr. Marotta is trying to understand if the person with whom he is working has a dream, acknowledged or secret. If he can find it and help it become a reality, that is fuel for the voyage and the foundation for hope. "My college professors were often priests who thought of life as a pilgrimage. My medical school psychiatry professors were all classical psychoanalysts who stressed the critical role of the creation of a meaningful life narrative." Part of the work is helping patients to understand that reality is always a combination of positive and negative experience, for example, recognizing that to get the benefit of a life-altering medicine you must accept the negative side effects. Understanding life as a journey and creating a life narrative that encompasses both the negative and positive is the evolving goal of treatment.

---

* Transference is a common occurrence between patients and team members. It is when either or both parties project feelings and emotions that are attached to past relationships onto the present one, thus clouding the ability to actually see things objectively.

The Door Is (Almost) Always Open

Rocky is working in his office with his associate Katharine; the door is open. A patient comes back from doing a blood draw across the road on campus and wanders into Rocky's office. Soon, they begin a conversation about his current response to a medication change. "Dr. Weiner, what do you think?" Rocky calls out to Howard (another team psychiatrist), who is also working with the door open across the hallway. Howard gets up and joins Rocky and his patient in Rocky's office and they discuss possible adjustments to handle some recent side effects. Meanwhile, Jackie (a senior social worker on the team) is walking nearby in the building, and on hearing this patient's voice puts her head in the doorway to say hello to him. It is a moment of spontaneous collaboration, one that is repeated often between staff and patients, staff and staff, patients and patients. It happens because both patients and staff feel safe.

The feeling of safety is both a physical and emotional experience. Sometimes you need the privacy afforded by a closed door in order to share experiences, but often feeling safe arises from an experience of unconditional connection and inclusion. Rocky's open door welcomes people to enter and connect, and it is fundamental to his nature to invite people in. In fact, Rocky thinks that SHH's campus encourages the collaborative interconnection that he believes is central to the work they do. Open doors, open spaces between buildings where people can walk and talk together, communal gathering spaces, all pull for a less fragmented and hierarchical experience within the community. "I was trained in an institution where doctors met patients in their private offices behind double closed doors to assure their privacy," says Rocky. "But I think that sometimes truths are more easily revealed in open interplays which are no less serious."

This physical door of Rocky's office that is almost always open, later becomes internalized by his patients as the connection that endures beyond their time at The Lodge. They (and their families) learn to trust that Rocky and/or others in their treatment team at The Lodge will be there for them as they move through their hospital experience into the future. "[The team here is a] very close-knit family," says Suma Srishaila, MD, one of the team psychiatrists. "When you have a caring, loving family, you can see it starts off with the values of the parents and their experiences and how they care for the family. Rocky's way of seeing our patients very much creates this dynamic because he sees our patients as family."

THE ROLE OF HUMOR

Walking down the hallway to Rocky's office, there are a couple of things most people notice. The first is that his door is almost always open unless he is in a patient session. The second is that infectious laughter often emanates from that small space. For Rocky, humor plays an important role in his interactions with both patients and their families. Unlike the neutral stance of more psychoanalytically oriented therapists, he wants patients to be grounded by a sense of connection to who he is and what he thinks. Sarcastic humor has no place in these interactions because he wants his patients to feel safe in his presence. Instead, gentle teasing or a joking nudge is a way to raise ideas, and to assess a patient's ability to think more abstractly and respond more flexibly. With all of his patients (and their families), Rocky is looking to build a sense of attachment that will be a tethering connection during the hard work of rebuilding their lives. If a patient can laugh at Rocky's jokes, he knows that they now understand the difference between an idea and a reality, and that relationships can be relaxed and enjoyable. Joking also allows him to show affection indirectly, without increasing anxiety in patients who are often frightened in the earlier stages of their illness by a more direct show of attachment. It is a shared moment which helps to build a relationship. And relationship is at the center of Rocky's success.

BEING AN ANCHOR

Rocky enjoys his patients' success openly and takes delight in helping when asked. He tells them all, "Take your medicine, stay sober, and watch who you date!" But like a grandfather, once they leave the program his presence mostly lives in the background, not the foreground of their lives. A number of patients, after a couple years of treatment, have gone back to school, and some to work. Many have transferred to transitional communities, are back home with their families, or are living on their own. Some call or text him every day; others wait for him to call. Some have clear insight into their progress and others have a limited sense of how much they have changed. Rocky celebrates them all. "What could be better than seeing someone do better?" he says. "It gives me great joy." What is true for all his patients, however, is that they know how much he cares. And the knowledge that he will be there no matter what, is a powerful lifeline. The winds and tides may ebb and flow, changing the immediacy or intensity of patient connection, but Rocky remains anchored. It is not unusual for him to reconnect with someone who has drifted away, returning months, even years later, following the rope pull of his periodic check-ins, just to see if they were okay. That is the power of enduring connection. It can pull you to safety if you are drowning. And, if loved ones are drifting, Rocky provides an anchor for families waiting for their return.

PUTTING IT ALL TOGETHER

We can sense the wheels turning in our readers' minds: Dr. Marotta sounds like an inspiring clinician, but how does that help those of us who have no access to The Lodge program and the work that he does? Our answer is this. While Rocky's style is unique, what has inspired trust in his patients, their families, and his staff are qualities that are not singular to one man and his mission. There are other psychiatrists, who, with their own style, bring caring and expertise to the work they do with their patients. For example, many of Rocky's colleagues have incorporated the approach shared in this book into their own outpatient work with patients. There are also networks of clinicians dedicated to reimagining and rebuilding the lives of individuals with NBD, who share ideas and referrals with each other across the country.

Look for a psychiatrist who is open to listening and respectful of the opinions of others, who is invested in thorough evaluations and flexible in their approach to medication. Look for a clinician who is committed to sustaining relationships with their patients and believes that stabilization is only the first stage of progress toward building a meaningful sense of self for their patient. Search for someone who would be open to the ideas presented in this book because they are always thinking about the process and what else can be done. Ideally, find someone who is connected to a community that supports their work. The techniques presented in this chapter can be useful to anyone interacting with someone struggling with NBD. Here are some of the key ideas of Rocky's approach.

KEY IDEAS FOR CHAPTER TWO:
THE CAPTAIN

- Core approach: the general principle is that what is to be treated is a constellation of symptoms, not a diagnosis. Think about underlying systems issues that may be contributing to the symptom picture.

- Look at individual case history: failure to achieve results in the past is seen as a source of information not defeat, a waypoint on the path to success.

- Out-of-the-box thinking: try creative approaches to persistent problems; consider using medications that may not typically be used with psychotic illness that might be possible interventions for presenting symptoms.

- Find a way in: searching for points of commonality is the first step toward building a relationship with a patient and their family.

- Maintain connection with the patient and family: this involves numerous strategies that may include being "sneaky," being perplexed, and engaging the patient through humor. It often involves playing different roles, including becoming a cheerleader, a life coach, and a mentor/teacher. It also involves leaving the door—to an office or to communication—(almost) always open so that people feel welcome, safe, and supported.

- Involve the patient in their own treatment: try to understand if the patient has a dream, either acknowledged or secret. If the dream can be found, clinicians can collaborate with their patients to help it become a reality. The dream can become fuel for the voyage and the foundation for hope.

- Encourage rehearsal of normal behavior: even if it precedes insight, rehearsal of normal behavior is important. Creating a virtuous cycle where one positive behavior stimulates other positive behaviors is part of the movement toward a happier life.

"The Wizard"
—A Parent's Story

The Right Kind of Connections

The precise details of our story have blurred, probably in the interest of self-preservation; to relive the exact date, time and places spanning over twenty-five years would make for a very precise but clinical tale, devoid of the human aspect. And humanity is precisely the point—without it, this would be simply a listing of diagnoses, doctors, and doses, without context. What we need to tell is the story of heartbreak, a Wizard, and creativity—ending in happiness.

The Dark Ages (1992–2013)

When we became a family of three in 1992, J. and I certainly thought we had it all figured out. We would balance careers, parenthood, and an active lifestyle. Those were the societal expectations, according to everyone—so they had to be real. Or so we thought.

Our daughter was everything—and more. Luminous, happy, energetic. We commuted and had a live-in nanny. All the right boxes checked. *What to Expect* became a joke book—and we discarded it.

But various milestones didn't occur by any book. Speech was slow to develop, then came in torrents; eye contact was random at best. We sought professionals for advice. The result was head shaking, shoulder shrugging, and random ideas: "She's gifted!"; "She's an only child!"; "You're a career mom!" Ironically, the nonprofessionals (i.e., friends and family) supplied the very same responses.

There was no question: our daughter was intellectually talented, socially reserved, highly creative. She was also joyful and exuberant. A talented writer and an avid reader. In 2000, I had left my career and reinvented as a stay-at-home mom to a private-schooler (much more difficult than any position I had previously held). Other mothers and I organized the usual play dates, carpools, and activities—and, if not perfect, all seemed okay and surely not worrisome.

But as preadolescence loomed in the mid-2000s, life grew intense and tumultuous; despite our daughter's continued strong academic achievement, we saw personal turmoil within. We tried and failed to reach her as

Continued ➤

we always had, but it was as if a wall had arisen. The temperature under our roof rose dramatically. Again, we sought resources, and again, our worries were downplayed ("She's bright, and highly sensitive!"). By 2010, the idea of an early college program up in the Berkshires—as she exclaimed, "Finally, these are my people!"—was exhilarating for all. We were actually exuberant at the thought of distance, a disturbing admission, then and now.

No book could warn us about the impending flood from an apparently dodgy gene pool. Unknown to us, it was vast and murky. Who held this responsibility? Each family kept the secret stories and facts yet resisted full disclosure. To this day, the vaults lie unopened. We are not big fans of looking back—too painful, and now, very much beside the point.

Those first few months of college were tense, and we had a local psychologist engaged by 2011. Still no commitments to diagnoses beyond "bright." A few antidepressants were tried, with minimal results.

THE FALL

And then, fall of 2013—more aptly named "The Fall." Our daughter was granted a gracious "leave of absence" from a second college experience, and we pursued drug and alcohol treatment at a facility that had been recommended by the psychologist. This had been a truly jarring development. We didn't (or wouldn't?) see that self-medicating had become our daughter's new hobby. The stay was short-lived. We received a phone call after one week stating, "this is bigger than us," to please "come get your daughter," and "you might want to read up on psychotic disorders."

Here was our family, just over twenty years after we began. What did this all boil down to? Tears, anger, fear—individually, collectively. What do we do? All we could do was listen to Tom Petty on the long ride down Route 7. Maybe Tom could help. No one else seemed to be able to connect us to a solution.

We were scrambling for ideas on next steps, while the three of us tried to coexist under one roof again. The local psychologist suggested we consider high level treatment, at least starting with a consultation. Her recommendation was Silver Hill Hospital. Ironically, we were already aware of Silver Hill from our own Fairfield County youth: "the Hill" loomed large for teens who occasionally drove past the facility ("That's where the celebrities go!"; "Don't make eye contact—they'll bring you in!"). To consider this step truly forced some reckoning with where we were now. Nudged

Continued ➤

forward by a friend, a Silver Hill alumnus who explained the programs and humanized the old images for us, we initiated admission.

What we didn't know—about everything—was stunning. Our internal chaos matched that of our daughter, and the three of us were each a mess. While still shell shocked, we met solicitous staff and spent a weekend in a "Family Session." Our daughter adjusted to a new version of "dorm living" and "group sessions." We tried to regroup. Our lives had changed abruptly. Forget conventionality, expectations. They're out. And maybe that's a good thing. But we were all lost, for different reasons.

Halfway through the twenty-eight-day program, Dr. Tom Landino did a phone interview with J. and I prior to a neuropsychiatric evaluation. Forty pages and an ink bottle later, we had a cauldron of labels to consider, each in the cul-de-sac of psychotic disorders. Finally, concrete but terrifying evidence: exhibits A–Z. Our twenty-eight days ended in December. But we were back at Silver Hill in early January, this time to the Acute Care Unit, after the psychosis presented itself as a truly unwanted Christmas gift.

2014: The Year of the Wizard

During that holiday season, the true gift to our family was Dr. Rocco Marotta. We felt an immediate sense of relief: Dr. Marotta—we were encouraged to call him Rocky—exuded assurance and empathy, decisiveness with a creative outlook. He spoke of treating the symptoms, not labels. We were shocked that such a human, and esteemed expert, could exist.

Our daughter was introduced to clozapine in the ACU, and we held our breath. We also requested that this be an "open-ended stay," until we could all see, and agree upon, actual progress.

Upon discharge some three months later, and while attending successive intensive outpatient programs, our daughter worked with Rocky in individual treatment. She was able to complete her degree locally, while enduring the side effects of clozapine, although now supported by the stimulant Nuvigil. She was stabilizing, but still under a cloud. Truthfully, none of us were quite sure what stability would look like. Had we ever experienced it?

Our daughter tried a variety of local volunteer opportunities as an effort to engage again. While the medications were certainly improving her capability and outlook on life, we could all feel the underlying dysfunc-

Continued ➤

tion and worked to accept the new reality. A few additional off-label medications were tried during this time to offset any other physical/emotional issues that arose. This was trial and error, resulting in a truly customized regimen. Meanwhile, our family was rebuilding, slowly. We were courteous and kind with one another, respectful of boundaries and limitations. We behaved as if we were on one long diplomatic mission. And our collective well-being relied upon knowing that we had the support of ever-present Rocky, whom we now affectionately referred to as "The Wizard."

The "Great Aha"

In the spring of 2016, Rocky raised the idea of incorporating Oxytocin into an ever-expanding regimen. Again, déjà vu—wasn't it a maternity drug? Rocky explained the essence of the hormone and its ability to encourage social engagement, connectedness, and more. The "aha" was clear: these were indeed symptoms that could bear treatment in our case, and we were all on board very quickly. As we made clear, at this stage we had nothing to lose.

Over the next few years, independent living [for our daughter] came along slowly, evolving from a local sober house with roommates to solo apartments in close range. No matter the location, we were heavily involved and supported every effort. This in itself was a great learning experience for all, and not without its missteps and frustrations. We were certainly a long way from the two college experiences in 2010 and 2013.

A New Old Life

Throughout, we were fortunate to be able to agree on one thing: we were a team (and if we didn't always agree, we kept working at it until we did). Our daughter was an adult but wanted to improve her quality of life; she was determined to comply with all treatments in order to regain her chance to start again. We stood together, as one—a favorite Tom Petty declaration.

We were all starting over in every sense of the word. Our daughter engaged in more varied and longer-term commitments to nonprofit volunteer opportunities, and we saw a gradual, growing aptitude for engagement with us, with others, and with a few select longtime friends who had remained in her orbit throughout her journey.

We recognized real progress when our daughter became restless to "really get going"—to create the life she had missed out on and truly

Continued ➤

could imagine now. Evidently, we had hit stability—and more. We were witnessing the reincarnation of our young girl as an adult, with wit, personality, intellect, and joy reclaimed. She chose to enter a graduate writing program in 2021, leading to a master's degree two years later in May 2023. While a student, she created and nurtured peer and mentor relationships in a way we could never have imagined in the days "Before the Wizard."

And as our daughter was thriving, so was Rocky and The Center for the Treatment and Study of Neuropsychiatric Disorders at Silver Hill. We became aware of it when we decided, as a family, that we were now capable of reaching out to others beyond ourselves. As parents, we had lagged behind our daughter's stability. But once our veil of grief had lifted, we knew that it was time. It was as if the oxytocin was in full effect all around.

Silver Hill and The Center have, quite simply, saved our lives. And we are hopeful that the "Oxytocin Effect" might become contagious, encouraging further steps toward peer support and outreach to those who need us. With our success comes responsibility to help others, and we take this very seriously.

Our daughter has launched a career in writing for non-profits. More significantly, she speaks freely and objectively about her experiences, including the emotions felt along the way. She plans to offer peer support when the opportunities arise and is adept at conveying the importance of medication.

We don't know what the future holds—we do know that there is no cure for these psychotic illnesses. We have hope—and that is enough for us. This entire process required a leap of faith—and a commitment to medication. These are not easy or convenient, but have certainly proven non-negotiable.

Rocky has given us success through a creative combination of traditional medications and one special hormone to treat our daughter's symptoms. That sounds like a modern-day fairy tale, but fortunately, we have a Wizard to guide us!

Chapter 3

THE CREW

"Book [knowledge] will not qualify you for [this] position. It's
personal. It's something that has to be in you. I don't know exactly
what to call it, but it comes from the inside. If it's not from the inside,
you couldn't do it."

—*Curtina Alexander, LPCA, Senior Residential Counselor, The Lodge*

The spacious common room at The Lodge is empty except for Sidney, a
large, overweight and balding man in his early thirties who is alternately
lying on the sofa and getting up to pace. The large television over the
fireplace is not on, the room is quiet, but Sidney is air boxing an unseen
opponent. Not so unusually, the tiny staff room, connected and open to
the common room, can barely contain the four team members: a doctor,
a social worker, a residential counselor, and a nurse, who are packed like
sardines, two sitting and two standing. One is on the phone, another on
the computer, all are discussing how to get another resident to an emergency medical consult—his blood work has concerned them this morning.
There is a shared intensity of focus, back-and-forth conversation, and a
joining of minds that are comfortable working in sync. And just as quickly
as they came together, the team members disperse when the consult is
arranged. This was an unscheduled meeting on an intensely scheduled
day. There are individual patients to see, groups to run, Rounds to make,
notes to write.

Sidney is still pacing, and Curtina Alexander, Senior RC, joins him at the counter. They stand, heads bowed together. Not much talking, just a moment of eye contact, but more than he tolerated when he first arrived. There is a gentleness to her manner, an ability to take her cue from what Sidney needs and can tolerate. And that little change in eye contact is noted and will be celebrated later when the team is rounding on all the patients.

It is time to introduce you to the Lodge's team, the crew whose skill is essential to the navigation of this ship. Their ability to help the passengers settle in and become receptive to the help that is offered is the central hub of the program. While they often look to their captain for consultation and inspiration, it is the skill of their day-to-day work with patients that allows the ship to move forward and this important leg of the NBD journey to take place.

THE LODGE STAFF IN ACTION

COMPASSION AND HOPE

It bears repeating: the staff members at The Lodge love their patients. They are psychiatrists, social workers, residential counselors, and nurses whose ethnic and racial backgrounds are diverse, ages wide-ranging, and pathways to professional life remarkably different. But they have a few things in common, the first of which is that they all chose to work with this population. The second is that they have each embraced Dr. Marotta's core approach. Many of them have seniority in their fields. They have been drawn to The Lodge program because of their belief in the underlying philosophy, and, like Dr. Marotta, their sense of connection to their patients is nonjudgmental and noncontingent. They believe they can help their patients attain more satisfying lives, and their hope is contagious and not limited by diagnosis. Each resident is valued and nurtured for who they are at each stage of the voyage, rather than only for their potential. Staff celebrate one second more of eye contact with a resident as excitedly as their ability to participate in a group.

Team members walk a fine line between maintaining hope and managing expectations, and they look to each other for the support they need to keep their balance. Each individual brings to the team an expertise informed by their unique history and training. One is a psychoanalyst, another did her foundational training in a different culture, another started her professional life working as an ER technician, and still another was a lawyer before changing fields to become a nurse. Every staff member has a moving story of how they were drawn to work in this field, and that journey gives them a unique window and perspective that strengthens the team.

TEAMWORK

Therapeutic work at The Lodge does not only occur at a set time in an office. All interactions between team members and residents are considered part of the treatment process and occur at all hours of the day and evening. Rigid ideology has no place in the team's work. Many of the team draw on personal experiences when thinking about their patients, and education, professional experience, and formal and informal conversations among team members play significant roles in staff decisions. Team process is not hierarchical. Each team member contributes to treatment formulation and then respects the ultimate decision that must be made by whoever is primary therapist on a case.*

Cases are constantly reviewed and reevaluated, allowing treatment plans to be reformulated with the addition of new information and perspectives. There is a complex organization of checks, counterchecks, procedures, and sign-offs designed to minimize risk while allowing the team to make decisions that may go beyond conventional conservative procedures. If a resident's primary doctor is not at the hospital when a crisis occurs, the team works collaboratively to step in and address the issue, communicating with the doctor as necessary and possible. There is no "your patient" versus "my patient" perspective at The Lodge, and team members do not stop thinking about their cases when they leave at the end of their shift. It is not unusual for staff on one shift to check in with the staff

---

* While the team process is not hierarchical, the team respects that the ultimate legal responsibility for each case resides with the psychiatrist who is primary on the case. There is real and substantial morbidity and mortality associated with NBD, both in the process of the illness and in unintended consequences of treatment. Medications have side effects and a patient may have occult and dangerous vulnerabilities below the surface. Treatment is dependent on very technical knowledge, which is constantly being reevaluated and modified. Someone must be held responsible, and that is the physician of record and the medical and nursing staff.

on another, or to call each other before their next workday with thoughts about a case.

Dr. Marotta puts it this way: "The team are people who over the years have become attracted to each other in some way, trust each other, and the process. I think of them as being a bunch of saints. They are people totally committed to the caring of others." The team members put it more succinctly: "We are puzzle pieces that fit."

CHEERLEADING

The staff at The Lodge see their job as cheerleaders who are fundamental to the process of their patients' sustained recovery. Part of the devastating nature of NBD is the revolving-door experience of so many patients and their families. If you set out on a voyage and hit repeated reefs and sand-bars, necessitating return after return to port, at a certain point you will get wary that you can ever make your way. "Is it even possible?" you might ask. "Why try?" The answer is that to continue, you need hope that it is not only possible but worth the effort. And as you near or bump into each obstacle, you need to feel trust in your captain and crew, that they know how to steer clear and keep going.

Cheerleading is important because it fuels resilience. The Lodge staff has had the benefit of seeing significant change in patients occur over time, and their cheerleading is a genuine expression of hopefulness born of that history. Convincing patients to stay the course and not leave the program prematurely is easier if you have seen progress happen again and again, if you have seen medication and therapeutic interventions result in signifi-cant and positive change. But the timing of all interactions is important, and this is where the experience of the team is critical. The interaction between a patient and a staff member is nuanced, involving the ebb and flow, the push and pull, of support *and* challenge.

At each stage of the journey, team members work carefully not to overwhelm a patient's defenses, while gently challenging them to increase the social awareness and connection necessary to live a more purposeful life. The goal is always to help patients regain their ability to work and to form relationships, but this will look different for different patients and takes place over a significant period of time. It is part of the treatment team's job to help patients and their families figure out what a meaningful life looks like for them and how to best achieve it. One person may go back to school, get a professional job, and live independently, while another may need more support and less demanding employment. Some may be able to find partners in love, others will be satisfied with friendship or community connection. It is also the staff's job to help patients and their families recognize how slowly some change may occur. When illness has been long-standing, the brain needs time to heal.

RESPECTING LOSS, CELEBRATING GAINS, EMBRACING *WABI-SABI*

Establishing what the goal of treatment should be for a resident is an important part of the team process, and managing expectations is part of the journey. If you have no expectations, you have no wind in your sails. If you have unrealistic expectations, you are capsized by storms along the way. For families, coming to terms with what your loved one may or may not achieve, grieving the loss of fantasies you may have had, is a necessary development as a family collaborates with the team to support their loved one's life once they are discharged from the program. This is hard, and some families feel guilty around their sense of disappointment and wonder if they could have changed the outcome if they had done something differently. But the Japanese aesthetic philosophy of *wabi-sabi* helps us to understand there is great value to be found in the unfolding character of all things, in each of our voyages. It is the mission of the team to help both patients and families find this value.

Wabi-sabi encourages us to find beauty in imperfection. The word *wabi* means "a feeling of sadness and anxiousness from a wish unfulfilled... an acceptance of plans going awry." *Sabi* means an ability to find beauty and value in the imperfect character of the natural world as things deteriorate over time.[1] In many ways it has relevance to the voyage of someone with NBD and their family, and the teachings of The Lodge team.

Most of us have heard the aphorism about parenthood: "You are only as happy as your least happy child." While that is certainly simplistic, it gets at an important point. Most parents want their children to be happy, and this fundamental desire drives their behavior. Unhappiness, both for loved ones and their families, is often the consequence of unmet expectations or having no expectations at all. "A parent has to grieve their expectations and has to find a way to accept their child as their child, even if they're not going to achieve X, Y, or Z," says Howard Weiner, MD, one of the team psychiatrists. This is particularly difficult if you are grieving something that is intangible, like a loss of cognitive and emotional functioning, an "ambiguous loss."[2]

But letting go of early expectations and fantasies about what makes for a conventionally successful life is necessary for an appreciation of a newly charted life to grow. The process of reemergence from destabilization for each patient is equally and uniquely challenging in this regard. Not all individuals can regain their previous level of functioning, either because cognitive shifts have occurred or vulnerability to stress is overly disruptive. There is grace that comes in recognizing the tremendous courage, strength, and work that it takes to accept this loss while celebrating one's gains. There is a deep healing and peace that can be found with the acceptance of the life we are actually living. Reformulating expectations is an essential part of creating a purposeful and satisfying life. Resilience, says Dr. Pauline Boss, a pioneer in the field of loss and grief, is not forgetting one set of experiences in order to replace them with another, but rather tolerating and accepting the ambiguities of life over which we have no control.

Helping a resident and their family identify goals that will support success rather than invite failure is critical. It is part of the mission of the team that patients and families do not give up because they feel defeated. They know that resilience, and the growth that it fuels, is central to the process of recovery.

ROUNDS: THE ART OF COURSE CORRECTION*

Whenever a new staff member or intern first meets with Dr. Marotta, he will always insist that they join in the weekly Rounds to really get a sense of "what we do." One outsider confessed that when she heard this, she walked

---

* In the context of medicine, *rounds* refers to the physician and other health-care professionals reviewing a group of patients. In a hospital setting, *rounds* refers to how doctors will typically go from bed to bed, observing and discussing patients' symptoms and progress.

over to The Lodge at the appropriate time, imagining that she would be walking around the building seeing patients at bedside, only to find the core staff were nowhere to be found. She walked back to Dr. Marotta's office and, knocking on his door, found the tiny office filled with a total of eleven staff members, some on chairs, one standing, and one on the floor against the closed door. Everyone was huddled together, with Dr. Marotta at his desk with the computer open to a patient's medical charts, alongside a Microsoft Teams virtual meeting window that included three more people attending online. This was Rounds!

Once a week, in a meeting that lasts anywhere from an hour to ninety minutes, all those who work in a significant way with patients at The Lodge (from Admissions to the pharmacy technician to the nurses, social workers, psychiatrists, and student interns and fellows) join Dr. Marotta in his office for a team meeting. Rocky is inclusive and welcomes anyone on staff to be a part of these meetings as he mentors his team and attempts to help patients in the most comprehensive way possible. While the meeting typically starts at ten o'clock in the morning, it is not uncommon for some of the staff to come down earlier, as they relish the premeeting conversations, that could be about anything from current politics to Greek mythology, dance, music, and popular culture. There is always laughter and joy and connection among staff during these treasured moments.

Rounds is the place where each patient at The Lodge is discussed in great depth. The attending psychiatrist and social worker will begin by giving a general outline and update. Current medications will be discussed, and recent lab work may be described. The residential counselors, nursing staff, and any other team members might add their observations from interactions that they have had during the week. Emails or phone conversations with family members will be described, patient involvement and participation in groups are considered, along with behavior in the general milieu of The Lodge and roommate dynamics.

Dr. Marotta uses his phone to call a colleague or consultant as he hears about an unusual symptom in a patient and tries to brainstorm it during the meeting; he asks his research assistant to look up an article to confirm a suspicion; he thrives on the intimacy of a team working together for the good of each patient. Unburdened by filling out forms, the team can go "round and round," revisiting issues. A general picture will emerge. The team will then discuss how they see the patient improving, possible medication titrations, augmentations, or changes.

Are they missing something? Will an MRI, EEG, or additional blood work be able to show a causal path that has not yet been considered? Maybe this will not change the treatment protocol, but it could give a greater understanding of the etiology of the illness. For Dr. Marotta, it is always imperative that treatment remains focused on the individual, not a diagnosis. He guides the team to think outside of the box, to find what will work specifically for each individual case. This is the magic of true collaboration.

Let's listen in on a typical discussion between the staff during rounds. It can give us some insight into both the philosophical and diagnostic approach the team takes to patient care. Here are some comments from different team members about various patients:

"His eyes are sometimes softer. The poor kid is suffering. He is being tortured. If this was the second century AD, he would be a saint fighting with the devil; fighting with demons in the desert."

"Grooming better; laughing more. On a nice load of clozapine. Things are going right. A lot of progress. Not held captive in the same way."

"Ever since oxytocin, doing more, talking, playing piano. Yesterday he ended the day by playing softly. That's significant. Taking in other people's needs."

"As psychosis loosens, not only is internal biochemistry off, but the recognition of damage to self and people around them increases. This is very common and dangerous. Hopelessness and despair and feelings they can never be forgiven.... Worried about her suicidality.... Everyone needs to be very watchful. Her shame is very loud right now; I have my worry radar up on her."

"Let's think. Given the erotic craziness, getting her more related with oxytocin might backfire. Are we driving mania with anything? Maybe lower lamotrigine.... There's good data for haloperidol being antimanic."

"Something about her metabolism that's tricky. Something about the particulars of her illness that all the conventional [medications] don't touch. Could be some strange genetic variant. Maybe not a specific illness, but something to do with her liver is hampering our med combos."

"He is a lot better!"

"What did you do?"

"I didn't do anything, just followed the 'magic' protocol! ... In addition to schizophrenia, he has a profound attachment disorder. So maybe oxytocin was exactly what he needed. He was a quick responder to the oxytocin. Standing straighter, more movement in facial expression, sleeping a lot later."

"Another with huge spike protein—antibody against Covid. She's had it some time or she's hyperimmune to the vaccine. She is in range with clozapine. Say we thought Covid was part of the picture, what would we add...? The Covid epidemic is changing the clinical course in a number of ways."

"She feels protected by delusions because she is able to surrender to God."

Go slow, give it time. Holding on to delusions suggests she's had them for a very long time. They must be holding something important together.

What are some of the take-aways from these fragments of conversation?

Fundamental to their work is the staff's compassion for the suffering of The Lodge patients and the staff's ability to bring different perspectives to an understanding and interpretation of patient symptoms. Rounds is one of the moments when shared professional and personal experience, intellectual curiosity, and book knowledge provide the fertile soil for evolving treatment plans and nourishing the professionals whose dedication to the mission of the program takes enormous psychological energy. Dr. Marotta's interest in history and mythology encourages others to engage a wide lens when thinking about patients' internal battles and how to help them to develop a meaningful life narrative.

Discussions are thought-provoking, with everyone given a seat at the proverbial table. Team members value Dr. Marotta's leadership and they look to him for guidance and contributing thoughts. But they also know that he will think carefully about different perspectives from his own. This delicate balance between respect for individual experience and the belief in collaborative problem-solving allows staff members to feel empowered but remain connected at the same time. Dr. Weiner says it succinctly:

What makes The Lodge team process special is the nature of the relationships among the team members. Throughout the staff, there is an attitude of respect and affection. We are able to share ideas openly and to challenge one another in a safe and supportive context. We are all willing to extend ourselves for one another. The feeling of this connection enables all of us to explore new ways of doing things. We are empowered to attempt different approaches without the fear of criticism. This ethos helps each of us to feel that we are never alone in facing the formidable challenges of treating some of the most difficult situations in psychiatry.

Attention to medical details, past and present, is critical. Dr. Marotta and his team are persistent in their investigations into the impact of physical problems on psychological functioning and the effects physical issues may have on the success of prescribed psychiatric medications. It cannot be overstated: attention to possible underlying physical issues that may be impacting a resident's mental state is critical to the development of an appropriate treatment plan. If someone's metabolism is abnormally slow or fast, for example, it will affect the rate of medication absorption. An infection may exacerbate psychotic symptoms. Medically induced symptoms can mimic psychotic illness. If such physical issues exist and are not identified, no psychiatric interventions will work as they should. Residents undergo frequent blood work and other medical tests when they are part of The Lodge program. The team appreciates that this is not easy. Nor is keeping track of and following up on the details of a patient's history. Contemporary administrative control and reimbursement policies hinder the work, while producing lots of required documentation. Also, patients are not necessarily forthcoming with accurate information, especially early in the process. The "truths" reveal themselves over time, and not necessarily in the doctor's office. That is why it is so important to have time to be with the patients, and time for the staff to communicate with each other.

Time for medications to "cook." There is hardly a Rounds that does not include someone in the team suggesting that a particular patient needs "time to cook." This has nothing to do with actual cooking but rather refers to the process of allowing a medication enough time to work. Experience in this field and with this population has repeatedly shown that a particular medication regime may not have immediate results. Furthermore, clozapine in particular requires careful titration over weeks and months. Hence, the patient and treatment team need to allow for this time as the medication achieves its full potential for a given individual.

A big advantage of The Lodge's long-term residential program is that it provides the space and support for patients to "cook"—and hence for the treatment team to truly observe whether or not a particular medication regime is effective. In the view of the team, it is a critical failure that so often sufficient time is not made available, leading to a limited use of clozapine and the unnecessary suffering of patients, families, and communities in our country.

Communication among staff, who see patients in different contexts, is the foundation to putting together the puzzle. Addressing the constellation of patient symptoms is enhanced by different perspectives and the ability of all staff to actively listen to each other. This kind of active listening helps staff to further distinguish personality characteristics from their patients' psychotic defenses. Often those patients who are getting better are still hiding some piece of their inner struggles, and while decreasing overt symptomatology drives initial interventions, the importance of a resident's past experience and personality organization become increasingly important factors in understanding what they can regain and how they can be reintegrated into normal experience. "I've just been so impressed by the interactions between having a psychotic illness, but that you also still have your underlying personality there, which is also going to reflect on your behavior," says Dr. Weiner. Identifying the psychodynamic and transferential elements of each case, when they become clearer, is an important part of staff discussion, as is the importance of attending to both staff and patient group process during moments of community instability. The ability to communicate a wider perspective is often a teaching moment for less experienced staff. Staff-to-staff support, as well as staff-to-patient support, is an important factor in The Lodge's smooth functioning.

A protocol is seen as an initial guiding structure but not as a rigid path. Each patient is treated individually, and each medication prescribed, adjusted, stopped, or exchanged according to a patient's symptoms and the medication's underlying affect and attendant side effects. While clozapine is the most effective antipsychotic for treatment-resistant schizophrenia (see Part II of Chapter Five, "The Importance of Medication and Sobriety in Recovery"), some patients have difficulty tolerating its side effects and other medications are considered. And while oxytocin has been a remarkable addition for many patients, for an "eroticized craziness," it might not make the most sense! All of The Lodge patients end up with a highly individualized treatment plan, and this regimen gets reevaluated with regularity. It is understood that smooth sailing, while celebrated, is never guaranteed. It is unusual for a long voyage to be entirely smooth, even in the best of circumstances.

PUTTING IT ALL TOGETHER

Putting together a team of people to work with someone with NBD takes enormous time and energy. Often, individuals' inpatient experience is short and their referral to post-hospital care is poorly integrated with their inpatient treatment. Care is easily fragmented, and this makes developing and sustaining healing relationships difficult. While the key elements below are drawn from The Lodge's extended care experience and provide a guide when searching for other programs, many of these elements can be applied to creating a team of clinicians who will work together once your loved one is discharged from a hospital stay. Above all else, seek crew members who believe in the power of continued relationship in the treatment process.

KEY IDEAS FOR CHAPTER THREE:
THE CREW

Alongside the captain, the crew have a "ring-side seat to miracles." The crew is a team of psychiatrists, psychologists, social workers, residential counselors, and nurses. Their passion for the work and their expertise are central to the process of recovery.

- Core approach: a sense of connection to their patients that is nonjudgmental and noncontingent. The crew believes they can help their patients attain better lives, and their hope is contagious and not limited by diagnosis.

- A fine balance: the crew constantly maintains the balance between providing hope and managing expectations.

- Constant care: all interactions between the crew and patients are considered part of the treatment process and can occur outside of a 9:00 a.m. to 5:00 p.m. working day.

- Team process: every crew member is invited and expected to contribute to treatment formulation. It is a collaborative process and not a hierarchical one, though the crew respects the ultimate decision that must be made by whoever is the primary therapist on a case.

- Team roles: in addition to their areas of expertise, crew members see their job as compassionate cheerleaders; cheerleading is important because it fuels resilience.

- Identifying patient goals: the crew works to help patients and their families identify goals that will support success rather than invite failure.

- Remember through this difficult journey, the philosophy of *wabi-sabi*: there is beauty and joy to be found in imperfection.

Chapter 4

THE PASSENGERS

"It was as if someone had found a loose thread and slowly pulled it
over a few years until he completely unraveled."

—*Alum Parent (about their son)*

In our eyes, the individuals and their families who struggle with NBD are
heroes whose courage in the face of enormous odds is remarkable. They
have often had to captain and crew their own ship, but at The Lodge program they enter as passengers, placed under the care of an experienced
captain and crew for this piece of their NBD journey.

Families with loved ones suffering from NBD come aboard Silver Hill
Hospital at different stages in their voyage. For some, they have watched
their loved one weather the sea of this illness over decades, watching them
drowning, losing sight of them, picking them up in whatever lifeboat they
could access. For others, their loved one may have been a strong swimmer
early in life, even winning medals along the way, only to succumb to the
waters later on. For all these families, the journey has been an exhausting
one. They have tried repeatedly to bring a loved one to safety and help,
and vessels have often been broken, the crew unqualified or limited by
regulations, and the illness has ravaged on. They live with the constant
anxiety that while they are searching, their loved one may be lost to suicide or drug use, be exploited by others, or, ravaged by the illness and the
internal voices they cannot quiet, harm others themselves.

Typically, families hear about The Lodge program and call the hospital or Dr. Marotta personally, desperate to find a way in for their loved one. Some families will mortgage a house or draw on their retirement funds in order to finance this rescue, which is not typically fully covered by insurance. But finances may not be the only barrier they encounter. Getting their loved one to agree to treatment is itself not always an easy task.

On any given day, Dr. Marotta's phone will ring and there will be a desperate parent on the other end, explaining their situation. An adult son, in his twenties, has been using marijuana for some time, is delusional and paranoid, and refuses to believe he is ill. How can this parent help their son? Or it may be an adult daughter, hospitalized now for the tenth time, who is stuck in an emergency room and is refusing treatment.*

Dr. Marotta listens to these families tell their stories over the phone. For some, nothing short of a court order will get a seriously ill loved one on board. For others, there are consultants who might intervene and help. Still others will have to find a way to cajole their loved one to take this step. Many of these families will suffer several more storms before they can get their loved one on board, and Dr. Marotta knows that he may not hear from a family again for a long time. We at The Lodge all know the heartbreak of these situations.

This chapter focuses on the experience of the patients and families whose journey has led them to The Lodge program. Especially for family members, there is often an initial feeling of relief that they have found a sturdy boat for this leg of the journey. But adjusting to the uncertainties of a new environment takes courage and time. Especially for the residents, The Lodge approach to treatment can feel unfamiliar. Understanding how they and their families are integrated into the inner workings of The Lodge sheds light on the philosophy that drives this different approach to acute care.

---

* Many of those suffering from the most severe mental illnesses suffer from anosognosia, a neurological condition where the person has no insight into their own condition, as can happen in dementia and with brain lesions or some types of strokes. This significantly impacts a family's ability to secure help with adult loved ones, whose free rights are protected in the US and other societies, thereby allowing them to refuse treatment unless they are deemed a danger to themselves or others (see Chapter Seven: Denial of Illness).

RESIDENTS

When a loved one is finally brought to the program, they most often come on board via the ACU, where they can be monitored and their most acute hallucinations, delusions, and agitations addressed before they are transitioned to The Lodge. Let us think of the ACU as a kind of lifeboat, similar to a hospital emergency room, a first stage of rescue from drowning in deep waters. In the ACU, they are placed on starting doses of medication. Dr. Marotta and his team are very careful to ensure that a prospective Lodge patient has been stabilized sufficiently at the ACU before they begin their longer stay and treatment in The Lodge program. Given the complexity of psychiatric illness and the accompanying behavioral risks, medical staff speak of the constant pressure to accept transfers they feel are not stable enough for the environment of The Lodge. This pressure comes ultimately from the insurance companies that deny care on acute hospital units, requiring patients to be released prematurely.

The tension is real at times, and The Lodge team is lucky to be an integral part of a hospital setting that allows quick changes in treatment planning. This does not mean that residents will arrive at The Lodge free of their disordered thinking, but The Lodge, unlike the ACU, is not a locked unit, which although a "selling point" to help engage patients in the program, requires that they can go without constant supervision. While structured, it allows the residents much more freedom within that structure, and they need to be able to handle this environment before they arrive. During their stay at The Lodge, residents' medications will be titrated upward or changed and combined with other medications to address the full range of their symptoms. If necessary, a patient may move back and forth between the ACU and The Lodge during their treatment journey at SHH.

SYMPTOMS AND BEHAVIOR

Initially, when they arrive at The Lodge, patients display a variety of behaviors. Some residents are mute or withdrawn, some are angry or agitated, some confused, and almost all are uncomfortable and frightened. The staff expects the transition to The Lodge program to be a process, with no set timing, and are careful to tailor their approach to each resident according to what they see when that resident steps through the door. There is more freedom at The Lodge than patients have had in the ACU, but there are also rules. Residents are surrounded by some of their belongings but in an unfamiliar place. They do not have access to their cell phones or computers, so they can stay present and open to the therapeutic milieu and all programming. They need time to adjust and settle. They need time for the effects of medication to deepen and for their disordered thoughts to recede more fully. They need time to build relationships.

Building a relationship with patients requires gaining their trust. In order to assess medication side effects and parse out other physical issues from primary illness symptoms and personality characteristics, patients need to accept all the evaluation and blood work necessary for these questions to be answered. Only with this developing partnership will the team be able to truly understand whether or not a resident's aggressive demeanor reflects a continued defense against less visible remaining paranoia and fearfulness or is part of an underlying character structure, or whether a resident's withdrawn behavior reflects residual psychosis or underlying shyness. Time and trust make the difference between a more superficial diagnosis and a deeper level of understanding. "Neuropsychiatric brain disease patients are a very stigmatized population," says Curtina Alexander. "If I treat someone as nothing more than their diagnosis, then I'll never get their trust, never get them to where they need to go."

ADJUSTING TO MEDICATION, SIDE EFFECTS, AND THE PARTICULAR BURDEN OF CLOZAPINE

For most patients, there is a constant tension between wanting to feel in control of their own lives and accepting the need to take serious medications that inevitably come with significant side effects. For families in the midst of overwhelm, the desire for a resolution to their loved one's suffering can make tolerating the initial experience of medication side effects difficult. While encouraging patience during the process of working out side effects, the team takes complaints of side effects seriously. The issue of side effects is germane to all medications, and psychiatric medications are no exception.

Currently, there are no antipsychotic medications without any side effects at all. However, certain medications are more or less intense in their side effect profile. Clozapine, which is often the antipsychotic treatment of choice for those entering this program after multiple unsuccessful treatments on other medications, has some of the most serious side effects of all the antipsychotic medications. Especially in the beginning of treatment, patients who take clozapine may experience heavy sedation, drooling, dizziness, constipation, and weight gain. They must undergo weekly blood tests and constant physician monitoring to check for signs of infection and liver damage.[1] The team at The Lodge believes strongly that these side effects are worth clozapine's greater efficacy, however they recognize that without the necessary support, clozapine's side effects may be difficult for some residents to tolerate.

The benefit of being in a residential program with a supportive team during the beginning of medication management cannot be overstated. A significant part of weathering the side effects of medication is the collective support and cheerleading from experienced staff who have the knowledge and confidence to remind patients over and over again of why enduring these side effects is worth it. Each resident comes to the experience of taking medication with their own set of anxieties, personality characteristics, and disordered thinking. So, for example, while every resident taking clozapine is encouraged to help mitigate its side effects by getting daily exercise either at the hospital gym or walking the hospital campus, and vitamin supplements are generally prescribed to all patients once individual evaluation has taken place, the individual experience of each patient taking clozapine may be different and requires a sensitivity and specificity of response by the staff.

Some patients need to sleep more in the morning and are not forced to go to early morning blood draws. Some patients are put on additional medication to help increase alertness. The list goes on. It is important for residents to feel that their experience is acknowledged and that they have allies in addressing their struggle. It is also important, however, for residents to understand that the journey to better health often requires some discomfort. "Finding the best balance is the key," says Dr. Marotta. "I try to get my patients to be stoic, to both accept and overcome."

A resident gets support for tolerating side effects from a variety of staff in many different ways. Of course, the attentiveness of treating psychiatrists and primary therapists is essential, but in the early days of a resident's stay it may be the Residential Counselors who help them navigate through their feelings of sedation and lethargy and who report back to the rest of the team specific details about a resident's experience and ability to cope. The compassion of nursing and blood draw technicians is also a significant factor in countering discomfort, especially in the early stages of clozapine management. Nor should the importance of peers in this process be overlooked. It is easier to weather a storm if your fellow passengers model a calm determination to get better and an acceptance of side effects. In fact, as residents slowly settle into The Lodge community, peer modeling becomes a greater and greater factor in the recovery experience.

Peer Modeling

Gradually, as symptoms recede and contact is tolerated, residents slowly integrate into The Lodge community. They join communal meals, go to therapists' offices, and join groups. Importantly, in this kind of community-based program, patients who are further along in their recovery process become models for those who are just starting. They model medication compliance and social behavior. Friendships can develop, which often extend past program stays and into post-hospital life. Take William and Charlie, for example, whose blossoming friendship continues past their hospital discharge. Along with Jimmy—who frequently reminds Lodge residents attending a shared AA group to "Listen to the doc!"—they have supported each other's treatment compliance and continue to make considerable progress toward their individual post-hospital goals. Fostering peer relationships like this is seen as a valuable element in The Lodge's community-based model, as truly thriving outside the hospital means learning to live in a social world with connection to others. Dr. Marotta is always heartened when he is contacted by one patient who is concerned about another patient's welfare. The ideas of caring for another, and of mutually supporting and mentoring someone who needs your help, are fundamental to the community values practiced at The Lodge.

Staff members also model behavior to good effect. "Each resident comes in here in a different state," says Senior RC Alexander. "But when the residents can see you being kind to one of the most vulnerable people in the house, they follow what you do." The essential role of the Residential Counselor staff should not be underestimated. They are central to any therapeutic community and are not merely managers of the environment but the mediators of healing and a patient's return to the conventional world. They are the ropes and lines of the sailing ship that allow for the adjustment of course and the weathering of storms.

For some residents, change is more obvious and fast-moving. For others, change is subtle and slow. Speed does not necessarily predict outcome, as there are many variables at play in each patient's situation. What is critical for everyone, however, is developing the understanding that staying on medication is fundamental to sustaining long-term stability. Once a patient accepts this premise, their ability to make gains outside the program is predictably stronger. Getting peer support for taking their medication can be enormously helpful, especially during earlier phases when doctors are still titrating a patient's medication dosages and addressing side effects. Watching another resident who has already been through this and is doing well is a powerful element in the treatment: if someone you feel connected to in the program trusts their doctor, then maybe you should too.

Each of the residents have different stories and different symptoms, but they are connected by the common thread of their tremendous suffering. Over time, the effects of medication and living in a predictable and calm structure allow therapeutic alliances with the team and other residents to develop more fully. For example, Colin's progress over the fourteen months he stayed at The Lodge was only possible because the therapeutic alliance he made with staff allowed him to tolerate the long and arduous process of getting his medication regimen correct. Team members remember him repeating their counsel, "I know I need to be patient. I know this is going to take a long time," and repeating that he knew his "team" believed what they were doing was for the best. Over time, Colin internalized strategies aimed at helping him deal with side effects as well. The medication he was taking made him tired, but he made an effort to exercise and eat healthily. He would also talk about wanting to be "gregarious" and outgoing and have friends. These were reasons, he reminded himself and others, that he was sticking with the process.

Often, a breakthrough moment occurs when a patient can say to a staff member, "I am suffering. I do not know what to do." They are then more accepting and interested in modeled behavior. As they get better, patients are able to support each other in groups and through shared experiences in The Lodge community. As time passes, social interaction with strangers can be introduced, and ultimately, a readiness to practice life outside the hospital campus in other settings unfolds. This process takes place in small and measured steps, but it is an enormously important part of The Lodge experience.

FAMILIES

EMOTIONAL FORTITUDE

It is hard to be the family of someone with NBD, often incredibly hard. Many families have been forced to take on multiple roles as they try to formulate, advocate, and actualize a long-term plan to help their loved one who is struggling. There have been repeated "fresh starts," the need to normalize atypical experiences, the need to compartmentalize the different parts of their lives as they try to attend to their careers and parent their other children, all while they simultaneously struggle to prevent their loved one from repeatedly capsizing.

Too often, they feel ostracized or blamed for their loved one's illness and behavior, or their failure to succeed in conventional ways. Unfortunately, sometimes this comes from other families or providers. Other times, they must bear the rage of their loved one's paranoid fantasies while simultaneously trying to protect them and get them help. Their loved ones are frequently discharged too early, with inadequate follow-up care and too many limitations placed on getting them further or better treatment. This is accentuated by a medical care system that is focused on immediate containment—not cure or even care—as well as the excess focus in this culture on profit and efficiency.

Dr. Marotta has enormous appreciation for what the families of his patients have had to do before their entry into The Lodge. "I believe, the team believes, that one of the most critical things is that the family is involved in treatment," he says. "Most Lodge patients have been living with their illness for a long time, and while a sense of urgency usually surrounds their struggle, getting admitted to this program often requires patience and persistence, as does success."

Emotional fortitude must be present from the very beginning. "Someone has to be willing to call again, if I'm unavailable, and persist in trying to reach me and the staff, to hold me long enough to give me a narrative, enough to make me understand that their loved one's case is something I might be able to do a good job at," says Dr. Marotta.

Once their loved one is in the program, families need to trust the advice of the team, even if their loved one is resistant, which is not unusual in early phases of treatment. If medical workups are necessary, families need to agree and collaborate with the team. For many patients, it is critical, in the team's view, to address the possibility of complex physiological reasons behind the behavioral disruptions. For example, partial complex seizures may cause a patient to look depressed or psychotic, but conventional treatment focused on these symptoms will fail as it misses the underlying physiological cause. There are other cases of autoimmune disease, neuroendocrine disease, and even hydrocephalus that have been missed when clinicians have not done a deeper physical work-up. And always, in our society, there is the issue of substance use, and how it can induce and exaggerate the most severe neuropsychiatric disturbances.

Consequently, it is essential to keep an open mind to the possibility of missing something critical.* All of this takes time and relies on a family's emotional endurance alongside the courage of their loved one. Unlike some European countries, where extended stays and development of special programs are more easily funded, the kind of extended care given in The Lodge is not often significantly reimbursed by insurance companies, and so also imposes a heavy financial burden on the family. Time, stability of environment, and community are central to rebuilding a fragmented life. Thus, a family's ability and willingness to take on the burden of supporting these factors is an advantage in the recovery process.

COLLABORATION

Paying attention to the emotional well-being of families is seen as an important element in a patient's recovery. The dynamic between a family and their loved one who is intermittently or persistently psychotic has had a long and complex evolution. Carers seek to protect their loved ones, whose thinking and behavior involves an alternative reality, and direct them toward a more consensual view of the world through a variety of interventions. This involves enormous emotional and sometimes physical energy.

Initially, at The Lodge program, families are given respite from their primary caregiver role. Instead, they are afforded the role of passenger to give them some relief from the experience of having attempted to navigate, steer, and captain this type of voyage. Staff reach out to family weekly and are available informally throughout their loved one's stay. "I first try to put some kind of comfort in the parent," says Curtina Alexander, "because if

---

* In medicine, the bias of the first assessment and diagnosis often follows a patient throughout their treatment.

the parent is anxious and uneasy, then the child is going to pick up on that and immediately they become uneasy." Lodge families know all the staff and have access to them via telephone and email. "We make it our business to leave that door open for them. I had a parent tell me that this is the first place that their child has been that they ever got to just be parents. Their child had been sick for a very long time, so I couldn't imagine what that could be like for them."

Helping family members understand the reality of their loved one's illness is one of the more difficult jobs for The Lodge staff. "Understanding this reality often involves accepting a sense of loss," stated one team member. In a world filled with instant gratification, says Alexander, it is also difficult for some families to have patience. She also notes, "And when a parent doesn't trust you, it doesn't mean that you're not doing it right; it just means that they are afraid." To understand this takes more than book knowledge. Many of the team have loved ones with some form of NBD, and these experiences allow for a degree of compassion with families that goes well beyond what you learn in school.

HAVING PATIENCE

In the initial phase of treatment, patients often need some space to adjust to routines and be stabilized. Some have developed paranoid fantasies about a parent or family members. Although understandable, a parent's impatience can be an obstacle to adjustment at The Lodge. "Just for those first few weeks, while we're still getting through the worst of the side effects, it's easy for a loved one to say, 'Oh, this isn't working. My child is not happy. It's been four weeks now,'" says Elaina Cardascia, one of the Residential Counselors, adding, "And it *has* been a month, but just hang in there!" There is also the frequent complaint that the staff is not doing enough: "My child is bored" or "My son needs more therapy." But it is not always so clear what is really needed. The kind of change the team is looking for often occurs slowly and subtly, with multiple shifts in medication and therapeutic interventions.

When families are understanding and supportive of the team's objectives, the path forward is generally smoother. The actual navigation of a ship at sea is unlike that in a video game or a Hollywood movie. Real life, with real people who have been suffering injuries, physical and emotional, means that changing course—i.e., changing brain chemistry, changing intrapsychic structures—is more often a slow-moving process, with complicated turns and unforeseen turbulence.

As families build their patience and trust in the team, they learn the complexity of the process, the importance of time, and the way that their loved one's particular treatment protocol will be most effective. Some medications may be removed while others are trialed as the brain adjusts, reacts, and becomes stabilized. It may take months to achieve the shift that the team is hoping for, and family support and trust in the process is critical. Along with titration of medications, the team will also be helping therapeutically as a patient builds basic living skills. There is nothing simple about the process of building back a life torn apart by NBD. One of the most important gifts a family can give a loved one is the gift of time and patience that allows that process to be successful. However, we understand these gifts, even when freely given, are not without real costs to those involved.

GAINING A SUPPORTIVE COMMUNITY

Bringing together families and extending resources is important, and Dr. Marotta is not afraid to pitch ideas to families or to provide outreach to communities working with NBD. It is easy to feel alone in your struggle, and finding a supportive community where you feel understood and share emotional energy can be the source of inner strength and inspiration.

Some Lodge alum mothers have been connected to each other by informal networking, and some have become part of support groups, dubbed The Warrior Moms,[2] sharing experiences and helping to gather resources and connections that will help their loved ones as they reintegrate into life outside the hospital. There are alumni who are available to mentor discharged residents in AA, and families whose loved ones live together once they graduate from the program and are ready to live independently. Whenever possible, patients and their families are referred to communities that support families struggling with NBD, and there is supportive networking among these programs, scattered around the US and staffed by skilled and accomplished practitioners.

At so many different levels, having a sense of relationship to others who are in your corner is part of the healing process. Finding a doctor you trust and who you know will always captain the ship, a crew of team members who will implement the structure of treatment, trusting there are lifeboats waiting in case your loved one goes overboard, and knowing there are other passengers on this journey by your side are all part of what makes for a tolerable voyage. Just as patients further along in the program can help those who have just begun, families further along in this journey can help those who have less experience, giving emotional comfort and sharing advice. Families, as well as patients, often keep in touch with Dr. Marotta and the staff well beyond their Lodge stay, reflecting the depth of relationships that have been built. Hope is founded on what happens in the program, and in the knowledge that going forward there will always be someone by your side.

PUTTING IT ALL TOGETHER

Simply put, we believe that every patient with NBD should be defined by more than their diagnosis. Each individual should be evaluated for their own set of problems, and have goals developed to meet their individual needs and dreams of a meaningful life. At The Lodge, while the majority of residents are young adult males, they vary widely in their symptom presentation, their temperaments and personalities, and their lived experiences. This, of course, is true for individuals outside of The Lodge program as well. What is our message? Try to find programs that demonstrate a compassionate recognition that each of their patients is different. And remember, although there may be times when families must take on the role of a captain navigating the ship, they are also passengers on this voyage, deserving guidance and the support of others. Following are some key ideas from The Lodge program's approach to patients and their families.

KEY IDEAS FOR CHAPTER FOUR:
THE PASSENGERS

Sailing toward hope optimally involves bringing both those with NBD and their primary caregivers and family members on board the treatment program.

PATIENTS

- It is always critical to find a treatment program that will conduct a full patient evaluation that explores underlying physical issues that can mimic or exacerbate psychotic symptoms. If necessary, the program should be willing to collaborate with outside consultants.

- Patients need the gift of time on board in order to develop:
  - trusting relationships with the captain and crew (psychiatrists, social workers, nurses, residential counselors, etc.).
  - relationships with peers on board so that peer modeling can occur.

FAMILIES

- Family involvement is critical to NBD recovery. Family members are also considered passengers on this voyage.

- Families need to have the patience to trust in the process and be involved in frequent communication with the treatment team.

- Families' education about the illness is a key component of the recovery process.

- Families, as well as patients, need community (peer) support.

"A Thread Unraveled"
—A Parent's Story

Sometime during the Spring of 2009, our tenderhearted, fun-loving son went from being a popular student athlete to an isolated, edgy, suspicious stranger lost in his own thoughts. The light was gone from his eyes. He was unable to sleep at night, and I couldn't wake him for school in the morning. He skipped lacrosse practice and paced furiously in our backyard, talking to himself and gesturing oddly. In hindsight, I recognize what—earlier on—may have been prodromal symptoms. But as a family, we had no idea what was in store for us and for him. It was as if someone had found a loose thread and slowly pulled it over a few years until he completely unraveled.

I remember a call from the yearbook advisor asking me to pick up the photos I had submitted for his senior page; a family Christmas photo, our three dressed in their Sunday best, arms intertwined and laughing; a photo of him scoring a winning goal; handsome in a tux with his date and friends in a pre-junior prom group shot in our backyard; a panoramic picture, lined up with all his cousins on our lake house dock. Happier days.

As I waited nervously at a red light in front of his high school, a caravan of buses pulled out of the driveway. Windows open, green and gold pom-poms and streamers and cheering voices, I watched his senior class headed for graduation. Our son would not walk across the stage that day. His diploma would be mailed to us weeks later. He was locked in a crowded behavioral health hospital, likely splayed on a cot in a hoody and athletic shorts, strings removed, facing the wall, afraid and tormented by voices. Pulling over on the side of the road, I cried for twenty minutes. Emotionally exhausted, feeling isolated, confused and afraid, it was the first time I had allowed myself to grieve the loss of the life we had hoped for him.

The next thirteen years were a roller coaster of twenty-six hospital-izations, and in and out of an overflowing handful of programs and residential treatment centers around the country. As his parents, we did our best to educate ourselves on what we eventually learned was the onset of mental illness. After many interventions over the years, it became apparent that our son was living with serious and persistent mental illness.

I read everything I could find on the subject. Bibliotherapy was my only solace. I reached out to psychiatrists quoted in books, researchers

Continued ➤

mentioned in footnotes, NIMH, TAC, and NAMI, looking for answers and support. The few local psychiatrists, therapists, and counselors in our sterile suburban town were not experienced in the treatment of serious mental illness. In fact, both his pediatrician and our son's therapist, who had treated him for ADHD, thought his issues were a result of substance abuse. No one saw what we saw in the privacy of our home. Indeed, he had been drinking to excess at times and had begun to use marijuana. But something else was going on. We didn't know if the substance use caused the behaviors we were seeing or if he was trying to self-medicate.

The stigma of mental illness and the lack of guidance and support had left us feeling isolated and desperate. We felt it important to remain strong and upbeat for our other two children, attending their school and athletic events, trying our best to cover for the chaos my husband and I were trying to navigate at home. I learned to compartmentalize my feelings. It was such a confusing, complicated, and painful time.

He was bounced from program to program, and the social workers advised us he needed a higher level of care. Many of his hospitalizations were seventy-two-hour holds. He was involuntarily committed many times, depending which state housed his current program. Hospitalized, pumped up with meds, and released, over and over again, there was no continuity of care. I schlepped a big notebook with my handwritten medication history, symptoms, and outcomes from place to place to try to inform hospital staff. But often treatment providers just seemed to reinvent the wheel anyway as our calls to psychiatrists were left unreturned. HIPPA regulations prevented staff from talking to us and his records from being shared from place to place, and he was too paranoid to sign a release of information. His "rights" trumped ours as his parents, who were just trying to get him help.

I have since learned there are ways to try to navigate this broken system. But at the time, we felt powerless, as we had to move our son from placements in five different states throughout the country, taking with him the T-shirt quilt of his sports jerseys, which we hoped offered some comfort in strange and scary places and might help to keep him anchored to his past. The only peek we had into his inner world was a black speckled notebook where he scribbled disorganized thoughts, raps and the nonsensical sentences that clearly preoccupied him. We couldn't believe our loving son had become a stranger and that no one was able to help him.

Most programs would not accept him because he was too paranoid,

Continued ➤

noncompliant with medications, and not stable. He had to be stable to be accepted. But how and where could he be stabilized? A psychiatrist at a well-known behavioral health hospital told me he would take him in his psychotic disorders unit, which he described as "not the nicest place," and a back door into the state hospital system for the long term. My son was 19 years old.

After I completed yet another pile of paperwork and assembled documents, he was finally accepted to a program in New England. We drove him there to check in, only to be turned away by admissions upon arrival because he had become anxious and too manic for their milieu. I asked if we could get him in the nearby hospital to stabilize and then return. But our request was denied. They suggested I take him home and try to get him hospitalized there. I drove him the long nine hours home, while he laughed, bounced, cried, screamed, and tried to hug me while I was driving. I did not think we would ever make it home safely.

When we stopped at a fast-food restaurant to quickly run in to use the rest room, I scribbled a note and put it in my purse: "Please help me! My son is living with a mental illness. He is manic and needs to be in a hospital." When we crossed the state line, I planned to speed up and hoped to be stopped by a police officer and to give him my note. At home, I contacted the mental health mobile crisis team in our county. They were one of only two and could not commit to coming by our home for forty-eight hours. So, we once again relied on the police. As I write this, I don't know how we lived through those days. We were always on high alert and walking on eggshells. I can't even imagine how he was feeling.

Our son has a complicated illness. He is diagnosed with schizoaffective disorder, depressive type. But who really knows for sure? Over the years, he's been diagnosed by his doctor *du jour* with everything from ADHD, anxiety, major depression with psychotic features, bipolar disorder, schizophrenia, high-functioning autism spectrum disorder, among other things, and has been on dozens of different medications in different combinations. This is a story which is sadly likely familiar to other families like ours who have walked this walk with a loved one. Times have changed. It is now understood that addressing a first psychosis right away can positively affect the long-term outcome. But back in the day, it seems hospitals were less likely to diagnose a young person with this debilitating illness right away or perhaps to share this diagnosis with parents. I did not see the

Continued ➤

words "possible schizophrenia" or hear them until I was able to finally get a copy of his first hospitalization records years later.

He may have also suffered concussions during his years on the sports fields. On top of that, anosognosia, a lack of insight about his having a mental illness, made him challenging to treat and to parent. It took him many hospitalizations to develop the insight that medication helped him after having successfully "cheeked"* his meds for years. Then there was the allure of marijuana, which he was convinced was a balm for his ailing brain, but we now believe contributed to the onset of and eventual severity of his illness. He also had side effects that troubled him, compulsions like jumping, shadowboxing, huffing, and having to lay down on the ground. More meds were added on to deal with those side effects and those meds had their own side effects.

A few years ago, he went missing for ten days and was listed on a national vulnerable missing persons list. Police departments in the area where he was living as an outpatient were notified and a photo of him was circulated. We took his photo to bus stations and hospitals. We thought we had lost him, as he was gravely disabled and unable to care for himself. It was terrifying.

Finally, he called me at 4:30 a.m. from a hospital in a different state, over a thousand miles away from his last location, dehydrated, floridly psychotic, and with no memory of how he got there. He may have just been considered another runaway or another homeless young adult. But thankfully, someone saw him walking circles in their yard and called the police. A nurse agreed to talk to me on the phone. She said he had somehow lost a few teeth and he was crying and confused. She treated him and told me the hospital had no choice but to release him to the street. I pleaded with her to find him a bed in a psychiatric hospital and had to contact the police and his psychiatrist to convince them that he was a threat to himself or others to keep him safe until we could fly across the country and file for conservatorship. Without conservatorship in that state, our hands were tied, and they had no choice but to send him out the door to the city streets. Fortunately, our efforts proved fruitful.

A couple years before, I was advised I had to charge him with assault in order to get him the urgent care he needed. The police officers were the

---

* "Cheeking" medications refers to hiding your pills between your cheek and your gums avoiding swallowing them.

Continued ➤

best support we had. They understood and helped me play the system as they recognized our crisis. A mother should never have to sit across from her son in a hospital court and have to say she was afraid of him in order to get him the medical attention he deserved. I don't think either one of us will ever be able to forget the pain associated with that moment. I pictured him learning to ride his bike in our cul de sac and how he trusted me to steady him until he was able to do it on his own. Our relationship was fractured. In the mental health court, while filing for conservatorship, again I was forced to list his scary symptoms and inadequacies and to recount my fears in front of him, which was incredibly painful. From his perspective, I robbed him of his rights and just wanted to keep him in a locked facility. I know I hurt him terribly, and he didn't trust me again for many years.

Later, our son, who had been relatively stable at the time and living in a private group home across the country, contracted Covid in November of 2020. Although he did not have many physical symptoms, his mental health symptoms were hugely exacerbated. In the middle of a crisis, he was taken to an ER by the house manager and the director, who had come to know him well and did not recognize this completely out of control version of our son. Upon blood testing at admission, after waiting in a chaotic ER until the wee morning hours with a security guard at his side, it was discovered that his clozapine levels were dangerously high. His blood work also showed elevated white blood cells but with no sign of infection.

During pandemic times, we were not permitted to fly or to enter any hospital. His psychiatrist told us over the phone that he thought the sudden change in behavior was the progression of his illness and we should get him on a wait list—which was two years at the time—for a long-term locked unit for low-functioning patients. He told us a third of patients improved, a third remained the same, and a third worsened, and our son was likely in that bottom third.

So, our son spent six weeks in a hospital gown and paper slippers in a city psych ER without a proper room. No behavioral health hospital would offer him one of the few beds that became available because they claimed he was too high acuity and needed one-to-one care that they could not provide. Or he did not meet criteria because this was his new baseline and hospitalization would not improve his symptoms. His psychiatrist stopped returning our calls and emails and the psych ER was unable to reach him. We had no idea what to do.

Continued ➤

I pleaded with our insurance company to help. They assigned me a mental health case worker and urged me to somehow get him back to the East Coast when travel restrictions were lifted and take him to an ER and place him on a wait list for a state hospital. I trusted them. But I realized after climbing up their chain of command that they are essentially a business and our son's care was costing them too much money. Their consulting psychiatrist actually reminded me, "I am not your friend." They suggested my son be dropped at a homeless shelter and allow the county to take over.

The reality is that repeated hospitalizations are outrageously expensive. But if they covered aftercare in a residential treatment center—or any portion of it—expensive repeat hospitalizations may not be necessary for people like our son. Residential care for those living with other challenges, such as autism, intellectual challenges, traumatic brain injury, and eating disorders, are often covered by insurance. Our son is living with a brain disease. Why is serious mental illness considered differently? What about the Mental Health Parity Act?

I fielded a heated call from the medical director of the psych ER, telling me I had to find a place for our son or they would drop him off at a local unlocked board-and-care home. He said they could not keep him safe in this place, where the police brought handcuffed, dangerously manic people in regularly. They were an ER, not a hospital, and he was taking up a bed for too long. I remembered the tents of the young and homeless that lined the streets of a nearby beach and wondered if our son would end up there. A kind psychiatrist who saw the young man behind the illness tried to keep him in a solitary confinement room when it was available. She said he was not a candidate for a long-term locked unit. She suggested he needed a full neurological workup and was quite certain that Covid had affected his clozapine levels. But we could not get to him, and we had nowhere to take him. It's truly unbelievable that this all rested on our shoulders. The hospitals deemed him too acutely sick or needing one-to-one care they could not provide during the pandemic. Yet we, as parents, were expected to pick him up from across the country with nowhere to take him for help.

I wish we could rewind back to the time his symptoms began to surface. I wish we had known about Silver Hill Hospital. I wish we knew about Dr. Marotta and his team. The most important thing we ever did, for many reasons, was to reach out to Dr. Marotta and then to get our son to Silver Hill Hospital, and our family will always be grateful for that blessing.

Continued ➤

I am not a doctor, but even I suspected my son's amplified symptoms had something to do with the pandemic, inflammation, and the interaction of his medications. I knew him so well and none of this made sense. A mental health consultant who had become a friend urged me to join a new group of mothers he was assembling to help to support one another on weekly online meetings during the pandemic. Through those incredible connections, and [through] our sharing of resources in our new Warrior Moms group, I learned about Dr. Marotta and his team at Silver Hill.

I sent Dr. Marotta a marathon email explaining our situation and he replied! After a subsequent phone call, where he took the time to listen to our son's history for nearly an hour, he guided me through the process of how to get our son moved to Silver Hill with the help of a trusted colleague, a mental health advocate who would safely transport him.

When our son arrived, Dr. Marotta called right away. During a physical exam at admission, he and his colleagues discovered a life-threatening infection and sent him to a nearby hospital for immediate assessment and treatment. We believe this was just the beginning of how they saved his life.

Eventually, through stabilization in Silver Hill's Acute Care Unit and then transfer to The Lodge, under the careful and caring eyes of Dr. Marotta and his team, including Drs. Suma Srishaila and Howard Weiner, it was determined that our son had an autoimmune disorder that was exacerbating his symptoms. Dr. Marotta showed us a graph on his large computer of our son's blood concentration of clozapine and how it was inconsistent and affected by the infection. He was cautiously optimistic that he could help.

Dr. Marotta served as the contact point for our son's care, as he reached out to various colleagues and specialists to begin to put together the pieces of the puzzle that made up our son's illness. When we visited, he often invited us to sit in his office to chat about his progress, current events, history, and family. We have come to think of him as a cherished friend and advisor. Dr. Srishaila's warmth and empathetic support as well as her keen observations of our son's behavior was also something we had never experienced before.

Through our weekly calls with Jackie Ordoñez, his social worker, and often touching base with Curtina Alexander, the beloved Lodge house manager, who had become his most trusted friend and caregiver, Tom, the patient nurse, Kate and the most caring staff who came to know him well,

Continued ➤

we felt like part of the Silver Hill family. Our son had so many arms around him. We have never felt so supported and I know he felt the same way.

Due in part to the 24/7 observation of him for many months, they were able to fine tune his medications and to include supplements that all together have contributed to his noticeable improvement. It was a team effort led by Dr. Marotta and every single employee at Silver Hill, from the doctors to the nurses to the woman who helped to clean his room, everyone played a significant part in his recovery. Their compassionate care and kindness made him feel safe and the patience for and respect of our son bolstered his self-esteem and confidence.

Curtina was able to connect with him like no other and to earn his trust—no small feat—as they often danced to his favorite music, walked, and talked. She gently nudged him to pay attention to his grooming and hygiene. I also believe she helped pave the way to repairing and rebuilding our relationship with him. This was a precious gift. He seemed to realize all we had done for him was done out of love.

His advocate who had become our consultant was also part of his team, communicating regularly with staff, visiting and taking him out to lunch. Through his patience and gift in connecting with people, he also built a relationship with our son. Our son's sharp edges were softening, and we began to see glimpses of the young man we thought we had lost. The combination of time, the most expert medication management, understanding of contributing factors, as well as addressing those factors by consulting with specialists, and genuine tender loving care was the hallmark of his stay at The Lodge. The support we received from every member of the staff has helped us to heal as well.

Dr. Marotta communicated with us every step of the way, and there seemed to be constant communication between the members of our son's treatment team. Every observation, interaction, symptom was reported back and discussed until they had a complete picture of him. They did not try to change his behavior or to redirect him but instead allowed him to be himself.

Dr. Marotta's combination of clozapine and oxytocin seems to have addressed both his positive symptoms as well as his negative symptoms in a meaningful way. Several psychiatrists in the past had given up on our son, calling his illness treatment-resistant. Dr. Marotta would not give up on him. He searched for answers until he found them.

Continued ➤

Financially, on paper and at first glance, the cost of this care felt insurmountable. But when we consider what has been accomplished during the past ten months at Silver Hill and compare it to the seven-digit cost of the care we paid out-of-pocket over the past thirteen years, there is no question that his time at SH was worth every penny to our son and family. I only wish we had found it during his first psychotic episode.

After his time at Silver Hill, our son is finally on the road to his best self. He is still living with serious mental illness. But we have always hoped he would have purpose in his life, as well as joy, and to know he is loved. For the first time in thirteen years, we believe he may be able to sustain supported employment and live safely in a community outside of the long-term locked facility that we had previously been told was his only option. He is smiling again and so are we.

Although we are not able to turn back time and to erase all the past struggles, and we know there will likely be some bumps in the road ahead, we now have what I know will be an ongoing relationship with a most special place and people, who we know truly care about our son and our family. Dr. Marotta has called to check on our son's progress and I've had emails from his team. The most meaningful gift I can give to another family who is early on in this journey is to explore the opportunity for better days afforded by Dr. Marotta and the team at Silver Hill and to truly believe you are not alone and there is hope!

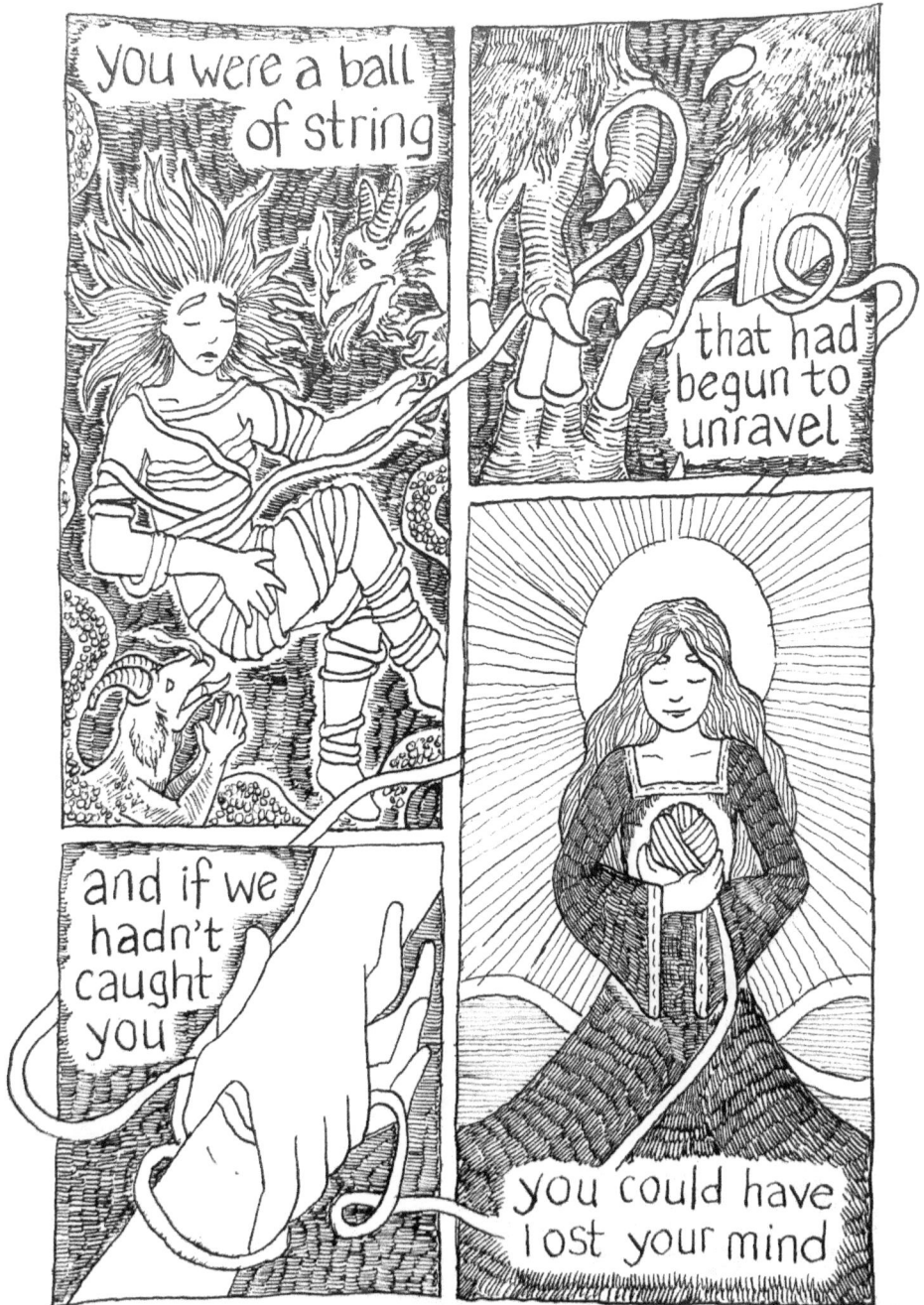

FIGURE 3: *Ball of string ink drawing*

Source: Permission to reprint from an artist who chooses to remain anonymous.

Chapter 5

THE LODGE VOYAGE

"If one does not know to which port one is sailing, no wind is favorable."
—Seneca

"They are ill discoverers that think there is no land, when they can see nothing but sea."
—Francis Bacon

The Lodge program is the beginning of a different kind of treatment voyage with a different kind of destination in mind. When patients and their families sign on to become passengers, they are signing on to a different kind of travel from that found in routine inpatient services or outpatient clinics. Reduction of overt symptoms such as hallucinations and delusions is only the first stop. Regaining a purposeful life—the ability to connect to the world and community, to love, to work—is considered the ultimate destination and marker of success.

There are three anchoring components to The Lodge treatment process:

1. Trust and relationship form the primary building block.
2. Medication and sobriety counter brain dysregulation and sustain stability.
3. A multifaceted treatment approach helps individuals to develop life skills, a sense of agency, and social experience.

PART I:
THE ROLE OF TRUST AND RELATIONSHIP

It might seem overly simple, but at the core of most successful, sustained outcomes for those struggling with NBD is the development of a strong, trusting relationship with at least one or more of their mental health providers. At The Lodge, our experience is that if a trusting relationship can be formed with even one staff member, a ripple effect will often occur over time, extending to the rest of the team and the institution. In this process, the alliances formed with families are often a critical bridge.

Before it is a conscious thought, trust is an unconscious experience. With roots in earliest life, it blossoms with positive acceptance, nurturance, predictability, and consistency of relationship. But it also requires that the person being nurtured is open to connection. Interference with connection abounds in NBD and consequently issues of trust are central to its treatment. These issues can begin early in life and are exacerbated by both the developing illness itself and the system that handles it poorly. The staff is aware that issues of trust exist both for patients and for their families.

Here are some of the factors that contribute to problems with trust and therefore with the development of relationship:

EARLY PROBLEMS WITH CONNECTION

Not all individuals with NBD show symptoms early in life, but many do. It is not unusual for families to report that their loved one was socially withdrawn, "always different," or was diagnosed with Autism Spectrum Disorder or Attention-Deficit/Hyperactivity Disorder, all of which involve difficulty with sustained connection. Perhaps their loved one doesn't like to be touched, or they can't sit still long enough to join in family discussions. Families who have been struggling to help their loved ones for years often experience repeated disappointments and setbacks. They have been trying to handle and treat these various conditions with no real sustained success. Their trust in mental health-care providers is already fragile by the time their loved one comes to The Lodge's program.

INTERFERENCE WITH CONNECTION FROM DISORDERS OF THINKING

Disorders of thinking often manifest in adolescence or young adulthood, although they may have had a secret presence earlier than that. Quirky behavior may have been interpreted by providers or family as boredom in school or a phase a child will "grow out of." Many health-care professionals shy away from diagnosing NBD early in a child's development, worrying about stigma or a family's angry reaction. Given a variety of possible diagnoses, families may, understandably, cling to the hopefulness attached to less serious diagnoses, failing to understand the serious implications of leaving NBD untreated. It is important to remember that psychiatric illness is a brain disease. We all understand that finding cancer at stage one rather than stage four can be the difference between life and death. Like any other physical illness, early correct diagnosis of NBD has a better prognosis.

Hidden disorders of thinking include paranoid ideation, hallucinations, delusions, and intrusive and confusing thoughts, all of which make connection to others and the development of trusting relationships enormously difficult. Thinking may be overly literal and sense of humor may be lost. Ideas may take on unintended emotional valence, may become too fast or fluid, or internal patterns of thought abruptly end. These processes make decision-making and interpersonal relationships very difficult.

For example, a young man with paranoid delusions and hallucinations may believe his mother has been replaced by a dangerous demon not to be trusted. This distorted fantasy obviously interferes with his ability to feel connected with his mother, but it also affects his mother, who no longer feels she knows her child. Or perhaps a young woman avoids contact with anyone because she believes she is a target of malicious intent. How can she make friends, connect with family, or go to school? How can anyone connect with her, no matter how hard they try, if she sees them as the enemy?

"Therapeutic alliance," the positive relationship between a therapist and their patient, is considered one of the most significant factors in successful treatment,[1] and requires trust in order to form. The team's ability to reduce disordered thinking and attention to internal stimuli in their patients is therefore one of the first tasks of treatment, as the success of the program depends on patients developing an ability to focus outward and then developing a therapeutic alliance with the treatment team. To this end, the team has to listen carefully and let the patients know they are taken seriously, but they must distinguish between constructive feedback and disordered thinking.

Some thoughts are intrinsic to a severely pathological delusional system—"This is not a hospital, it is a CIA prison" or "The doctors are demons, agents of the devil, or a malevolent government"—statements so bizarre that a diagnosis of schizophrenia is indicated and time on medication needed to resolve them. Or the accusations may be a bit less severe: "You are in it for the money"; "I am not really ill, but the hospital needs admissions to stay open"; "I admit I have problems, but this is not a good treatment for me"; "You do not understand me"; "You are not giving me enough treatment, time, therapy. . . ." The themes of "You are not doing enough" and "You are doing the wrong thing" are very common and are addressed with empathic listening and the support that allows for acknowledgment of changing perspective over time. Developing therapeutic alliances also requires the staff to recognize and acknowledge the multiple and complex psychodynamic elements, such as parent/child relationships, which get played out in this "extended family" setting.

CONTRIBUTIONS OF SYSTEMIC ISSUES

By the time they enter The Lodge program, residents and their families have almost all gone through repeated hospitalizations and interventions. Often discharges from hospitals and clinics have been premature, placing a Band-Aid on patient symptoms but rarely facilitating sustained recovery or changing core patterns of mistrust and anxiety that interfere with connection. In fact, these past experiences have often had the opposite effect, reinforcing feelings of betrayal by providers and mental health-care systems more responsive to regulations than common sense and the needs of the patient. Many of the patients have had very negative experiences with medications, medical staff, and police. These experiences have a profound impact on their ability to trust.

The often adversarial nature of our legal system, which keeps patients out of hospitals because they don't technically present a danger to self or others, is also problematic, as it delays appropriate intervention for an illness which becomes more fixed over time if it remains untreated. Our legal system is wedded to the principle of "autonomy" over "benevolence," even in situations where a patient's judgment is impaired by a brain disease that inhibits rational thinking. The Lodge program is predicated on a different vision of mental healthcare, but it takes time and early education for residents and their families to really absorb the difference and trust the staff. The Lodge team is willing to give it as much time as it takes. "We're just consistently there for them," says RC Cardascia. "We get to know them really well." Little moments beget bigger moments, and over time trust, connection, and autonomy grow. "For example, we ordered a resident's lunch for him and he was so excited. It was just a grilled cheese, but he was excited that we knew what he wanted, and he got it, and that made him happy. And then he went happily to group." This ripple or "butterfly effect" is at the heart of all successful treatment and depends on the development of trust between patients and the staff with whom they work.

PART II:
THE IMPORTANCE OF MEDICATION AND SOBRIETY IN RECOVERY

The vast majority of medical professionals have come to see NBD as a disorder of the nervous system, a brain disease, requiring careful treatment in which medications play a central role. It has also been long noted that the use of alcohol and other substances can play a role in the initiation and sustaining of aberrant behaviors. Therefore, helping our patients to understand the critical role of medication and sobriety in their sustained recovery is also at the center of The Lodge treatment. Understanding the history of how psychotic illness itself was understood and then formally diagnosed gives context to current medication interventions and considerations. For those readers less interested in the historical context provided, you may wish to jump ahead to the following section ("Current Perspectives and The Lodge Approach to Medication"), which describes the current program perspective on medication.

A Brief History of Antipsychotic Medications*

Premodern Psychiatric Treatment

To understand how psychotic illnesses, and specifically schizo-phrenia spectrum disorders, can be treated, it is helpful to look back to the earliest records of their recognition and description. There are references to what we would consider neuropsychiatric disorders in ancient literature, including the Babylonian, Egyptian, and Greek medical texts (the Hippocratic Corpus), as well as Indian and Chinese writings. What we would call states of depression ("melancholia" in the ancient texts), intoxication, agitation, confusion, delirium, and dementia are all described.

Disorders of behavior were thought to be caused by stress, curses, intervention of gods, alcohol use, dangerous environments, weather, or lack of proper education and discipline. While many thought that it was the heart, not the brain, that was at the center of thinking and behavior, even in ancient times there were some who taught that there was a relationship between the brain and behavioral change. For example, around 170 AD, the Roman physician Galen suggested the brain's four ventricles determined personality and bodily functions.[2] Throughout history, interestingly, various treatments were categorized, including exercise, travel, studying specific holy texts, eating specific foods and plants, drinking wine, using opiates, and, in India, drinking tea made of rauwolfia alkaloids (a class of drugs used to treat high blood pressure). Many of these and other interventions from the past continue to have therapeutic efficacy, which we now understand in biochemical terms. In our own time, diets, vitamins and supplements, exercise, and travel are touted as potential cures.

Over the millennium, an understanding of possible causes of "bizarre" behaviors gradually evolved, often within a religious

---

* The contents of this section evolved from an initial collaboration between Dr. Rocco Marotta and Dr. Suma Srishaila.

Continued ➤

and spiritual context. In the ancient world, people were treated in temples, and later in monasteries and religious institutions of various faiths around the world. Diet, quiet, and human understanding were always part of the equation. Unfortunately, outside of holy places, humane care was not a general rule. In the Early Middle Age, people with psychotic illnesses might be chained in asylums. Medications and potions were only partially effective, and there was always the risk of people becoming socially isolated, mistreated, and criminalized. No matter what the intervention, treatment response was not predictable, and a poor outcome was frequent.

A beacon in the history of early Western psychiatry is the work of Phillippe Pinel, who lived in France in the late 1700s. Among other things, he pioneered the removal of psychiatric patients from prisons and the medicalization of treatment of psychiatric illnesses. His efforts occurred in the context of the Age of Revolution and the birth of nation-states, who claimed to afford citizens or subjects new respect and consideration. Still, regarding the treatment of what were called mental disorders, there was a paucity of effective options. Throughout time, people have been frightened by individuals whose judgment, understanding, and communication abilities are impaired. Authorities often continued to be harsh in their handling of behaviorally aberrant or "mentally ill" persons, and in most settings those who suffered with these symptoms were separated from the rest of society.

Early in the nineteenth century, before the systematic development of medications, philanthropists, religious institutions, and some governments founded hospitals that were dedicated to treating mental patients in self-supporting communities. These "asylums" were generally institutions of safety for their patients, predicated on the idea that working within the hospital setting, exercising, and living in companionship with others was therapeutic.[3] As the nineteenth century developed, Western science and medicine, especially in Europe, became focused on understanding the physical causes of illness. The advance of chem-

Continued ➤

phrenias could be differentiated from those diagnosed with what were called the manic-depressive illnesses, even though both diseases might present with delusions, hallucinations, and disorders of thought and interpersonal connectedness. Those suffering from the schizophrenias showed a deterioration over time that had some of the qualities of dementia (hence Kraepelin's label, "dementia praecox"), while the manic-depressive illnesses cleared over time (although the process might be repeated). These clinicians predicted that, similarly to neuropathological damage to organs, each of these patterns would have a different underlying pathology and, therefore, would respond to specific treatment modalities. The hope was, and continues to be, that the underlying neuropathology of each of these disorders would and will lead to a more focused and effective plan of care.

Despite early hopes for a golden age of treatment, at the beginning of the twentieth century there were still limited knowledge and options to treat psychiatric disease states. These included rest, alcohol restriction, fresh air and a calm environment often found in the countryside, good food, and sedatives. In some areas of the Western world, other treatments were also attempted, including the use of opiates and barbiturates, with limited success. But only minor progress was made with treatment modalities other than attempts to provide more humane institutional care. In the 1930s, physical interventions that in our time may seem somewhat extreme began to be used. These included psychosurgery (e.g., lobotomy) and electroconvulsive treatment (ECT, which is still used effectively). This period, characterized by the expansion of cities, a marked increase in alcohol use, crime, and other social stresses, was correlated with an increase in behavioral disorders not unlike what is occurring now in the Western world. This resulted in pressure for hospitalization, treatment, and, unfortunately, imprisonment of people with neuropsychiatric brain diseases. Humane efforts were made to move large numbers of patients from cities to hospitals in the

Continued ➤

countryside. Nonetheless, despite the pressure on both medical and social policy to deal with the explosion of behavioral disorders, the great hope of transforming psychiatric care was not fulfilled. Separation and isolation of individuals rarely resulted in a positive outcome for those unfortunate individuals suffering from NBD.

The catastrophe of the Second World War ironically led to much technological innovation and some breakthroughs in psychiatric interventions. The war had resulted in great improvements in the treatment of trauma and of surgical techniques, however some patients who were felt to have undergone successful surgical procedures still died unexpectedly. It was thought that some of these deaths were due to hyperactivity of the nervous system, resulting in a type of autonomic nervous system shock. Consequently, a search began to find medications that would mitigate that risk. In the post-surgical wards in a French military hospital, Henri Marie Laborit, an army surgeon who had led the research teams exploring the calming effects of antihistamine medication, noted that a drug called promazine, a phenothiazine, was particularly effective. Agitated patients on this medication became calmer and more cooperative. Wondering if related compounds would also have a positive effect on agitated psychiatric patients, his team convinced colleagues in the department of psychiatry to evaluate the effect of these compounds on manic and psychotic patients. The result was unexpectedly good. After a slow start, in 1954 a landmark study, which was randomized and placebo-controlled, showed the effectiveness of chlorpromazine (Thorazine) in psychotic patients.

A promazine derivative, chlorpromazine is a member of a family of chemical structures called phenothiazine, which have had various uses historically (including aniline compounds used to dye expensive silk scarves). Organic chemists knew a great deal about these related compounds. However, the remarkable changes in behavior noted in psychiatric hospitals ultimately

Continued ➤

led to a revolution in psychiatric treatment. Many people suffering from severe psychotic disruption, including hallucinations and delusions, improved significantly when treated with compounds related to the phenothiazine structure, although they often became heavily sedated. These therapeutic successes, albeit rarely curative of the underlying illnesses, were of the greatest importance since they began a major shift in the medicinal chemistry of psychiatric and neurological treatment of psychotic states, depression, mania, anxiety, and movement disorders. Chlorpromazine's entrance into the market heralded the birth of neuropsychopharmacology.

Haloperidol, or Haldol as we commonly know it, was the next psychiatric breakthrough in 1958, and, like chlorpromazine, initially developed for other purposes. Janssen Pharmaceuticals was attempting to develop a more powerful pain medication (analgesic) and had identified this class of medications from the parent compound butyrophenones. They found it to be a poor analgesic; however, they noticed in experimental animal studies that it had similar properties to the phenothiazines. When tested on psychiatric patients, they noted haloperidol's clinical abilities to not only manage agitation but also decrease paranoia and delusions. Soon other medications structurally similar to Haldol followed—e.g., trifluoperazine, fluphenazine, along with the phenothiazines—giving clinicians and patients a spectrum of choices in antipsychotic treatment. These medications were called neuroleptics—"taking hold of the nerve"—and we now understand that they work by affecting neurotransmitter systems essential to the connectivity of the brain and the control of behavior. The dopamine hypothesis* was the most accepted theory about the causal root of schizophrenia, as it has been clearly demonstrated that a common mechanism in all of these first-generation neuroleptics or antipsychotic medications is the varying degrees of blockade in the dopamine receptors in the various pathways and

---

*The dopamine hypothesis posits that psychotic symptoms may be due to hyperactivity of a specific subset of the dopaminergic systems of the brain.

Continued ➤

regions of the brain which communicate with one another. However, there is consensus that the neurotransmitter mechanisms are nuanced and complex, and, in addition, show variance in each individual. Could a theory positing only one mechanism as the root cause of psychotic illness be correct?

This was a time of discovery, excitement and expectation in psychiatry, a field which had relied primarily on long-term psychoanalysis, institutionalization, ECT, and heavy sedation as the only available treatments for people who suffered from psychotic illness. Hope of cures and the alleviation of suffering, as well as expectations of cost savings from reduced psychiatric hospitalizations, filled the literature. This enthusiasm was soon tempered by a recognition of the dangerous side effects of these medications. It was a dilemma. Blocking dopamine, which occurred with these antipsychotic medications, was believed to be necessary for the effective treatment of psychotic symptoms. But blocking dopamine induced motor disorders, and for many patients still did not eliminate some of the most salient symptoms of the illness.

Serendipity continued to lead psychiatric intervention in positive directions. In 1958, just five years or so after the discovery of Thorazine, Wander Laboratory in Switzerland, while examining compounds known as tricyclics in their quest for new antidepressants, was surprised to discover a chemical structure which, while embodying aspects of tricyclic antidepressants, showed "neuroleptic" properties. One of the compounds in this series, named "clozapine," was especially significant as it was able to ameliorate psychosis without the disabling extrapyramidal side effects seen with Thorazine, Haldol, and similar medications. The psychiatric community was initially skeptical of this "atypical" antipsychotic (meaning psychotic without extrapyramidal side effects), as it was felt that medications which did not cause these side effects were unlikely to be effective in treating psychosis. Clozapine was less likely to cause motor side effects like Parkinsonism or dystonia, did not cause a rise in the hormone prolactin, and did not induce tardive dyskinesia. But its ability

Continued ➤

to reduce both positive and negative symptoms of schizophrenia spectrum disorders could not be denied. There was a problem, however. In Finland, clinical studies reported that a number of patients taking clozapine had developed agranulocytosis (a drop in white blood cells necessary for fighting infections) and eight patients taking clozapine had died. Nevertheless, physicians in Europe continued to use this medication carefully for treatment-resistant cases of NBD, with protocols developed to allow for early detection of changes in white blood cell levels. But in the US, it was taken off the general market and rarely used.

The Evidence in Support of Clozapine

Over the ensuing years, the data from Europe and Asia showed clozapine to be highly effective, and especially useful in treating severely ill psychiatric patients. Several large clinical trials in Europe and in the United States, including head-to-head trials with chlorpromazine, showed undeniably positive effects, and the pressure to reevaluate the use of clozapine in America increased.

Many other chemical compounds (e.g. olanzapine, quetiapine, lurasidone, risperidone) have been found to have antipsychotic properties and there has been increasing interest and focus on other receptors, including serotonin, GABA, and NMDA receptors, which might bring newer classes of medications into the market, hopefully with fewer side effects. But unfortunately, these medications—called "second generation neuroleptics or antipsychotics"—have not proved as effective as the older generation clozapine.

The later development of long-acting forms of medications, such as depot injectable Haldol, has had some noted success in treatment, since a medication that only requires acceptance once a month removes the daily struggle over compliance that leads to frequent rehospitalization of some patients (see Chapter Seven: Denial of Illness).

Continued ➤

At the time of this writing, a new medication, xanomeline/ trospium (Cobenfy), which stimulates muscarinic acetylcholin- ergic receptors in the central nervous system, has been released. It appears to be an effective antipsychotic medication with hope- fully a less troublesome side effect profile. We are now awaiting long-term studies of its efficacy or comparisons of its efficacy to that of clozapine with regard to persistent psychosis. This will allow us to make better decisions regarding individualized treat- ment plans.

Still, during the last decades, more and more data has rein- forced clozapine's reputation for being the most effective anti- psychotic, especially with patients who do not respond to other antipsychotic medications or have side effects when those medi- cations need to be used in higher doses. In 2015, a detailed pro- tocol called REMS (Clozapine Risk Evaluation and Mitigation Strategy) was developed in the United States to minimize the risk for patients placed on this medication, but treatment with this medication is still only encouraged as a last resort for indi- viduals who have undergone multiple unsuccessful treatments.* Outside of the United States, clozapine is used more regularly. It not only modulates acute psychotic symptoms but decreases rates of suicide (lithium is the only other medication that has been shown to do this), improves negative symptoms, decreases rates of readmission into psychiatric hospitals, has much lower rates of motor side effects, decreases the incidences of substance use, and decreases overall death rates compared to other medi- cations. Major studies have shown it to be more effective than any other antipsychotic medication.[4]

Why is clozapine still not used by many psychiatrists in the United States? Physicians who do not prescribe clozapine worry about the significant effects, including sedation, weight gain,

---

* As of February 24, 2025, the US Food and Drug Administration does not require prescribers, pharma- cies, and patients to report results of Absolute Neutrophil Count (ANC) blood tests before pharmacies dispense clozapine, as was required by the original REMS regulations. Physicians are still expected to monitor their patients.

Continued ➤

and risk of infection (agranulocytosis or myocarditis), especially in this post-Covid period where incidents of myocarditis have increased. Our adversarial legal system makes medical risk-taking of any sort a greater concern, while the administrative/regulatory aspect of using clozapine (REMS) has required a great deal of paperwork and expense. Additionally, patients may find the frequent blood tests to be a burden, and the positive changes that occur with clozapine can take months (and even years) to fully manifest.

But those psychiatrists who use clozapine with their patients have a very different perspective. While there is no question that some of the regulatory criteria connected to clozapine need to be revised, the intensity of staff-patient connection required when clozapine is prescribed is not necessarily negative. Following a patient closely while they are on this medication can be a specific and powerful way in which the treatment team can demonstrate their care and concern for their patient. This, combined with the miraculous therapeutic outcome which can occur at times, motivates physicians who use it. They are uniformly adamant in their belief that clozapine should not be the medication of last choice in the treatment of NBD, especially since the data suggests that the earlier psychosis is cleared and remediation is started, the better the long-term outcome.

For those wanting a more detailed understanding of the biological efficacy of clozapine, Dr. Lewis Opler's chapter in *Meaningful Recovery from Schizophrenia and Serious Mental Illness with Clozapine* (2017) provides an excellent synopsis, and *The Clozapine Handbook* by Jonathan M. Meyer, MD, and Stephen M. Stahl, MD, PhD (2020) provides a comprehensive overview. For our purposes, it is simply important to know that clozapine is the only antipsychotic medication that has a clear and consistent effect (over many studies) on the negative as well as positive symptoms of the disease. Because most of The Lodge patients have undergone multiple unsuccessful previous treatments, clozapine is often started early and, if tolerated, is the antipsychotic of choice. Dr. Marotta is a strong advocate of its earlier use and the need for changes in its overzealous regulation.

CURRENT PERSPECTIVES AND THE LODGE APPROACH TO MEDICATION

Over the last five generations of medical scientists and psychiatrists, biological research and technical progress in the area of neuropharmacology have led to an increasing understanding of the inherent complexity of neurotransmitters, receptors, and the interconnectivity of the brain. The relationship of these factors to cognition, learning, motor behavior, and emotional regulation suggests that a simple, unidimensional hypothesis about the underlying mechanism of schizophrenia related illnesses is implausible.

On a descriptive level, a diagnosis of schizophrenia has come to be accepted and codified in the *Diagnostic and Statistical Manual of Mental Disorders,* fifth revision (DSM-5-R), and the *International Classification of Diseases,* eleventh revision (ICD-11). This descriptive system derives from the work of many schools of thought and does not require the acceptance of a specific hypothesized underlying neuropathology or demand that the treating physician believe schizophrenia is a single existing entity. It is a paradigm of generally agreed upon criteria. The diagnosis exists as a best effort to help clinicians categorize and communicate among themselves, a diagnostic and cognitive "rubric" that states that Schizophrenia/Schizophrenia Spectrum Disorder (SSD) is characterized by symptoms that fall into three domains:

1. POSITIVE SYMPTOMS: i.e., experiences of distortion of perception (hallucinations), false or distorted beliefs (delusions), confused thinking, and disorganized speech. These are obvious presenting symptoms and have been studied in great detail. These are the symptoms that the conventional antipsychotic medications are most effective in ameliorating.

2. NEGATIVE SYMPTOMS: i.e., experiences of social withdrawal, lack of emotional expression, paucity of spontaneous movement, anhedonia (not seeming to take pleasure from life), lack of spontaneous speech. These are the symptoms that are less responsive to most antipsychotic medication. Clozapine is the exception.

3. COGNITIVE PROBLEMS: i.e., the experience or demonstration of difficulty with attention, verbal or nonverbal memory,

speed of information processing and executive functioning. An individual's IQ (a measure of "intelligence," as measured by standardized testing) may be less than expected, and some patients show a decline in functioning over the course of the illness; this led to the early descriptions of dementia praecox, or dementia of the young. Reversing cognitive decline is more difficult to treat and is often a major determinant of poor long-term outcomes. Different medications are used by The Lodge team to stimulate cognitive processes.

In reality, we know that patients suffering from NBD often have a plethora of problems that may not be easy to tease apart. For example, they may be suffering from a long-term, smoldering and progressive neurodevelopmental disorder that has interfered with their ability to learn or relate to others over a number of years. Or their illness may reflect an abrupt change in behavior, heralded by the onset of severe anxiety and paranoia, induced by trauma or drug use or traumatic brain injury. Perhaps they have an underlying genetic vulnerability or they were exposed to an extremely toxic medical trauma. There may be many and diverse paths that lead to a chronic psychotic illness like schizophrenia. "It would be naive," says Dr. Marotta, "to think that such a complex disorder, often the consequence of poorly understood genetic and biochemical processes, would succumb to simple interventions. When one works with young people suffering from NBD, you notice that they often:

- have high levels of overt anxiety

- have obsessive preoccupations

- are sad, depressed, and have been treated for depression

- are lonely and lost

- are dependent

- have a history of substance use, including cannabis, alcohol, amphetamines, and psychedelics

- have a history of learning disability, Attention-Deficit disorder, and other behavioral disorders such as conduct disorder and personality disorders

- have a higher rate of diagnosis of epilepsy

- have a history of negative effects of medication trials and early onset of side effects

- do not feel they have a problem or need help

- do not trust authority.

"Not only is the putative underlying substrate of NBD complex [e.g., disrupted dopaminergic and glutamine neurotransmitter systems, dysfunctional limbic system and orbital prefrontal cortex]," says Dr. Marotta, "but a developing brain may have greater vulnerability during certain periods of time. For example, during teenage years and a young adult's early twenties, the nervous system is undergoing extensive reorganization. It is also a period of accelerated learning and stress, and exposure to violence and cannabis or high dose stimulants during this period can have greater and long-standing consequences on a vulnerable brain. In fact, recent data supports the hypothesis that exposure to high potency cannabis during the teenage years seems to be resulting in increased emergency room visits for psychotic behavior, and also in the ultimate development of schizophrenia.[5, 6] Therefore, it is clear to our team that no single intervention, either psychopharmacological, social psychological, individual, or group based, will alone be enough. Everything must be evaluated for both positive, negative, and interacting effects."

Interacting elements must be considered. A model of care that is continuous, supports sobriety, treats anxiety and depression, resists the treatment for a single "diagnosis," and exists on multiple levels is critical. It is not enough to measure success by mere statistical change—by using, for example, the Positive and Negative Syndrome Scale for schizophrenia (PANSS), a quantitative assessment of psychosis—but rather by seeing an individual get a job, find friends, rejoin their family and community, and feel in their heart that they are worthy.

That is why a medical team treating such patients must often use a very complex medication regimen and must be vigilant not to make errors in diagnosis. For example, antipsychotic medications have different properties, which may be tried more or less successfully with different patients. Antidepressants may be added to treat resistant depressive symptoms. Lithium is frequently prescribed to address mood regulation, to help decrease impulsivity, and to help with maintenance of white blood cell counts for patients on clozapine. And when persistently resistant psychotic symptoms have failed to respond to other antipsychotic medications, clozapine becomes an important option. Even with the use of clozapine, however, residual negative symptoms may remain and interfere with maximizing functioning. At The Lodge, the addition of oxytocin has been helpful in further reducing negative symptoms. This is a relatively unique treatment strategy and one that deserves further elaboration. Let us take a closer look at this neuropeptide hormone, associated with maternal bonding and connection, which, alongside clozapine, is helping NBD patients make significant gains in the realm of social experience.

Oxytocin and the Quest to Facilitate Social/Emotional Experience

As in any long journey, the path toward the destination is often accomplished in stages. When dealing with acute psychotic states, the first leg of the voyage is the reduction of positive symptoms, allowing individuals to perceive experience through a less distorted lens, which, in turn, generally allows them to achieve greater stability of functioning. This kind of progress is often measured with quantitative assessments, such as the aforementioned Positive and Negative Syndrome Scale (PANSS), often considered the benchmark by insurance companies for release from hospital stays.

Once patients have reached technical criteria for discharge, however, many still face significant obstacles to reintegrating into more satisfying everyday experiences because their capacity for social/emotional connectedness is still significantly limited and limiting. Although they may no longer be hallucinating, they may continue to show poor focus or an inability to initiate action. Many spend hours before the TV watching sports or reruns or music videos, and lurking behind their often quiet and seemingly unemotional exterior, their minds and hearts are often suffering an extreme level of anxiety or a profound lack of psychic energy, which makes meaningful activity and social connection nearly impossible.

Over a fifteen-year period, Dr. Marotta and his colleagues have tried many interventions to potentiate the effects of antipsychotic medications and decrease these negative symptoms. These have included combining multiple antipsychotic medications, adding antidepressant medications, antiepileptic drugs, stimulants, cholinergic agonists, hormones, and ECT, among others. Mental health providers have developed therapeutic communities to increase support, help with socialization, prevent personal isolation, and help with medication compliance and sobriety, which are critical factors in long-term stability. But pharmacological interventions to address negative symptoms have been modest, at best, in their effectiveness. That was until Dr. Marotta began to add oxytocin, a neuroendocrine peptide that has been studied carefully for over thirty years, to the medication regimen of some of his patients.

Dr. Marotta began to add oxytocin to some of his patients' medication regimes about eight years ago. Why oxytocin? In his private practice, many of the forty patients on clozapine he had continued to follow were doing better than the typical NBD patient, going to school and work and staying relatively sober. However, they still exhibited some continuing signs of the illness. Many still showed social withdrawal and lack of motivation. They often lived at home with families or in isolated settings, were shy, were often able to articulate their desire for social contact but were very rejection-sensitive, and in general did not seem able to reach their full potential. An avid reader of diverse medical literature, Dr. Marotta had been reading about some interesting work using oxytocin with autistic children. Then, at The Lodge, he and the team encountered a case that ultimately reinforced his interest in oxytocin as an additional treatment intervention for patients with NBD.

Dr. Marotta and his team had a patient with a mild frontal lobe lesion and a long history of severe substance use—including opiates, cocaine, and cannabis—who continued to be withdrawn and lacking in social skills, despite over a year of complete sobriety and multiple trials of antidepressants. In trying to rethink what might help this young woman, Dr. Marotta considered that she might actually be exhibiting a syndrome of autism, and he was aware of the existence of a relatively small literature on the use of oxytocin to help in such cases. In both animal and human studies, oxytocin has been shown to have many interesting properties. The conventional psychiatric literature reflected a general suspicion about the usefulness of oxytocin in psychiatric interventions; the clinical data was "not persuasive." But Dr. Marotta was intrigued.

The human studies in the literature used an intranasal formulation of the drug, which Dr. Marotta felt would be inappropriate for his patient who had a serious history of substance use that involved intranasal drug ingestion. After going through whatever literature there was and concluding that it would not be a dangerous substance to try, Dr. Marotta and the team found a pharmacy that could formulate an oxytocin wafer that would dissolve under the tongue of their patient. A supply was acquired, and it was added to this specific patient's medication regime.

The team was surprised to see their patient improve quite remarkably over just a week with the addition of sublingual oxytocin. At that point she was being treated with bupropion, atomoxetine, and trazodone. When started on oxytocin, she had already been at Silver Hill Hospital, first in the ACU and then in a transitional living program, for over a year, and was still not well enough to return home. Notes from the medical charts document her own experience taking oxytocin: "I think it worked. Oxytocin helps. It helps me relate and be open with people. People find me friendly. I am less anxious, and I am now able to concentrate." Her family noted an enormous positive change. She was able to leave the hospital within a couple of months of starting oxytocin; she returned to college, graduated, went on to live on her own; she returned to her artwork. Eventually she was able to return to a high-level job, which demanded a great deal of interpersonal activity, and she continues to thrive with the addition of lamotrigine (Lamictal) to the aforementioned medications.

Initially, the team did not connect the results of this case to their work with schizophrenia spectrum patients. Instead, they waited to use oxytocin on the next autistic patient with a mild frontal lobe syndrome who would appear at Silver Hill Hospital. Fortunately, no such patient was admitted over the next many months, giving Dr. Marotta and the team time to think about how similar schizophrenic functioning can be to frontal lobe syndrome and related autistic behavior. In fact, one of the classic descriptions of schizophrenia, by the Swiss psychiatrist Eugen Bleuler, uses the term "autism" as one of the defining characteristics of the illness, along with problems of thinking, ambivalence, and lack of expressiveness. The team had many such patients and were continuing to admit them weekly. Dr. Marotta decided to give oxytocin a try. One of his colleagues provided a humorous reminiscence of that moment:

> Rocky and I would get into many fights about this because I am a dyed-in-the-wool statistician and, as by trade, a diagnostician. And Rocky is a brilliant psychiatrist and a dreamer. Rocky read about intranasal oxytocin for autism. And he said, "I like this. There's a lot of the same negative symp-

toms [between autism and NBD], a lot of motivational unrelatedness, social, emotional reciprocity issues." And he's like, "Let's do sublingual oxytocin for psychosis." And I said, "You can't just do that. You need to have a track record of demonstrative research!" And he's like, "No, we're just going to do it anyway." So, we did it ... and it was mind-boggling the difference, because I saw the patients, they would come to the office, and they were like night and day.

Since the published consensus was that, although not dangerous, oxytocin (given intranasally) was not an effective treatment for schizophrenia, initially it was decided to use it only with the most severely ill, unresponsive patients. These patients had already been on clozapine for at least a year, so any observed changes could reasonably be ascribed to oxytocin and not to the long-term use of clozapine alone. They continued to administer the medication in the sublingual form, as most of their patients had a history of serious substance use. Dr. Marotta and the team have come to believe that the significance of their results may have something to do with this alternative method of administration.*

Remarkable changes in some subjects provided an incentive to begin using oxytocin with a wider range of patients. Let's take the example of the young man who turned to his mother during a session with Dr. Marotta and complimented her cooking. Seeing her begin to cry, he seemed perplexed. "Why are you crying, Mom?" he asked. "Because you have never complimented my cooking before," she said. "But I have always liked your cooking!" he answered, not realizing that in his previously withdrawn state, he had never uttered his thoughts aloud. Or take the example of a teenager in the program, who, as a staff member recalls, "was very quiet and mopey . . . we had him for four or five months, and we got used to him being like that. And then once he started oxytocin, his whole personality came out in a way that we didn't even know it was there, and then watching his parents cry, because they were so excited the first time, they saw him. It was like he was there again, peeling off the layers and coming back out again. He made jokes all the time after that, he had friends, it was really nice."

---

* The team's hypothesis is that the sublingual mechanism of delivery may result in higher levels of oxytocin entering the bloodstream. This, in turn, may lead to higher concentrations of oxytocin delivered to the brain, or autonomic nervous system, or endocrine glands. This is one possible explanation for the comparatively better results to other oxytocin studies. Research focused on the delivery system is ongoing.

It is neither ironic nor strange that oxytocin, the neuropeptide hormone connected to bonding and love, should play a significant role in The Lodge team's positive treatment outcomes. While pharmacological intervention is essential to success, attachment is key to the whole process. Attaining and sustaining recovery is hard work. If you cannot grasp the hand held out to you when you are slipping overboard, it is exponentially more difficult to stay on the boat. Oxytocin, for a significant number of patients, helps that outreach to occur. It helps trust to blossom and decreases anxiety about connecting with other people. It consequently helps with family reconciliation and the ability to participate in community and make friends. It helps a sense of belonging to reemerge.

The result of this combination, clozapine and sublingual oxytocin, sometimes seems like magic, as Curtina Alexander enthusiastically noted:

> With the combination of medications together: Life! It looks like life. A lot of people when they walk in the door, it looks like life is just gone . . . and when the two medications start to work together you see them lifting their heads up, there is eye contact, there is literally socialization where they had stopped socializing. Like a person who has been here for months and one day they pick up the phone and they call their family. That's magic.

Elaina Cardascia, RC at The Lodge, describes: "They wake up, they make eye contact. They want to talk to me; they'll initiate the conversation instead of me dragging some words out of them. They'll go up to their peers and just be like, 'Is this your cheeseburger?' And we're all like, 'Oh my God, you noticed that person, and you spoke to them!'"

Often the changes are things that most of us take for granted, like opening a door, taking a shower and shaving, or playing the piano softly so as not to disturb other residents. One RC relates:

> I had one resident that went from using one-word answers to six words. It was reason to have a party. And we had one resident that wouldn't even go out the front door ever, and then one day I was sitting in the office, and they just walked out the front door, hugged me and said, "Thank you, C." Your heart drops and then the tears come right behind. We don't get to determine what a best self is, but our job is to help them get to where the best place is for now.

And Dr. Marotta observes:

> We see these changes as the beginning of virtuous cycles of change. Once you can make eye contact and then speak in a therapy group or an AA meeting, you have an essential skill that may allow you to return to school or eventually get a job. It may seem like a little thing, but it opens a door to reentering the world. Some of the patients tell me that their anxiety level decreases, and they can enter the social world. It is as if some pathological shyness begins to give way.

Interestingly, the impact of oxytocin can be subtle, and while some patients are conscious of its effect, some patients are less clear of the changes it triggers. The measure of its effectiveness, however, can be seen by those around them, who watch with awe as their loved ones who had been socially withdrawn and isolated for years become increasingly able to engage with others and articulate their thoughts.

Oxytocin seems to:

- decrease social anxiety

- increase the ability to articulate thoughts and feelings

- increase the ability to make and maintain eye contact

- increase cognitive capacity, in combination with clozapine

Oxytocin risks: none reported in the literature. The Silver Hill study of oxytocin paired with clozapine observed:

- no episodes of hyponatremia

- no tardive dyskinesia

- sporadic cases of abnormal liver function test results, which returned to normal

- sporadic cases of high eosinophils

- no cases of agranulocytosis

- no cases of myocarditis

- no onset of hypertension

- no sedation or excess salivation

The team feels the strength of empirical results warrants continuing use of oxytocin while research is ongoing, and the Center for the Treatment and Study of Neuropsychiatric Disorders is committed to pioneering research on the effects of oxytocin and the oxytocin-clozapine medication combination. Details of developing research projects can be found in the appendix.

The Importance of Ongoing Medication Adjustment

It is important to understand that clozapine and other antipsychotics do not generally cure psychotic illness but control it. Every stage of medication management is a fluid negotiation between a doctor, their patient, and the patient's family. As time and circumstances change, the need for medication adjustments (dosages, mix of medications needed to facilitate optimal functioning) frequently arises, and it is important that patients trust their doctor enough to remain in contact and hopefully accept their advice.

For example, over time original levels of medication may not continue to control voices completely, creating tension but not total dysfunction, or sedation or weight gain may feel so overwhelming that patients don't want to continue with medication at all. It is also not unusual, as many families know, for a patient who has been stable on medication for a significant period of time to decide that they are well enough to discontinue their medication despite advice to the contrary. This can be a heartbreaking and challenging experience for families, many of whom live with the anxiety that this moment will occur and now have to revisit earlier experiences of their loved one's dysfunction. At that moment it is ideal if a patient trusts someone enough to admit that they intend to change or stop taking their medication, and this information can be discussed with their doctor. Sometimes gentle persuasion or direct challenge can change the course of resistance and compromise can be achieved. But we all know that often the ideal is not the reality, and even if they try, a doctor can't overcome their patient's decision, despite their best efforts. However, if, despite this setback, they can maintain their relationship with their patient, their persistence may eventually be rewarded by greater acceptance of a compromise solution. At the very least, they will be available to help if their patient's boat capsizes.

What might this give and take between a doctor and their patient look like in this context?

- Continuing check-ins with a patient, e.g., "Are you okay? What's happening these days?"

- Listening and gently challenging distorted thinking, such as paranoia, denial, grandiosity, e.g., "Right now, something is off. You are not functioning at your best."

- Giving feedback about patterns of behavior, e.g., "It seems like every two weeks you get a migraine and feel more depressed."

- Focusing on dysfunction, which is more accessible and motivating to the patient, e.g., "Maybe raising your medicine will help you focus better in school."

- Telling the truth, e.g., "I fear for you." "I think things are going to go badly if you don't take your medication."

- Giving examples of patients who didn't take their medication and suffered tragic outcomes.

- Remaining outwardly calm despite provocative, challenging patient statements and behavior, but setting limits when necessary.

- Understanding that a patient may consider raising dosages, restarting medication, or returning to a hospital stay to adjust medication as a defeat, and therefore reframing the experience as an accomplishment.

- Collaborating with families and trying to create coordinated efforts and feedback.

On the positive side, Dr. Marotta notes that in the experience of The Lodge staff, many patients seem to require lower doses of clozapine after several years of treatment. This is especially true when they have had social and professional successes. "We view this as another example of the virtuous cycle of interaction," he says. "It is an example of learning and growth and making up for lost time."

The need for ongoing medication adjustment is yet another reason why patients who are able to have extended stays at The Lodge, or who return for a brief stay for a "tune-up" following discharge, develop greater stability. Real-world social environments encourage behavior that often leads to decompensation (the worsening of a patient's mental health condition), for example, the rampant use of substances such as Adderall, marijuana, and psychedelic drugs on college campuses. We exist in a culture that romanticizes free will and supports entitlement and desires to be special and admired, elements that pull vulnerable individuals toward unwise choices. Allowing for additional time surrounded by a supportive treatment team can help patients learn to tolerate side effects as they are being addressed over the course of many months and helps them to build the strength and resilience necessary to withstand the pull of dangerous social environments. Critically important, added time in the program helps patients come to a place of acceptance and understanding of the complexity of their illness and the critical role that medications and their treatment team play in their recovery. Once discharged from The Lodge, most patients need a longer-term residential placement where the skills they have begun to learn in the program can be practiced and the recognition of their own strengths and weaknesses can be solidified. Staying on their medication is key to sustaining gains and continuing to move forward during this next phase of treatment.

Does this mean that all alums of The Lodge stay the course and maintain their medication compliance? Of course not. The insidious nature of NBD, its seductive pull toward feeling they are not ill combined with certain personality profiles and temperaments, makes it challenging for some individuals to continue taking their medication consistently, especially when they feel better.

"Patients often don't want to disappoint us," Dr. Marotta muses, speaking about the not unusual ebb and flow of denial and confession that can occur when a patient goes off their medication. "They have often worked with therapists who are more dogmatic about following advice. We continue to work with patients even if they don't follow our suggestions, and over time they come to realize that we are not going to abandon them. This is a central part of how we develop trust."

Continuing contact with a patient's family, sharing information and giving advice, becomes very important in these situations. This is why Dr. Marotta and The Lodge team always request and encourage a patient to agree to have the team establish a family connection from the very beginning of a relationship. This allows an additional flow of information and collaboration to occur. No one is out of the loop and families can feel they have an ally in their ongoing struggle. No matter what, it is critical to hang on.

THE IMPORTANCE OF SOBRIETY

Historically, there are certain truths that are self-evident. One is that the excessive use of alcohol and substances can be dangerous. There may be a range of susceptibility to the negative effects, but data and empirical evidence have and continue to show that these risks do exist. In fact, there is an old dictum in Western medicine that any substance can become a poison; it depends on the dose and the susceptibility of the subject.

It is well known that excess use of alcohol can acutely lead to dis-inhibition, seizures, confusion, lack of judgment, and death, and it is no secret that many substances used both therapeutically and for "pleasure" (opiates, stimulants such as Ritalin, amphetamines, anti-anxiety medicines such as Xanax, Klonopin, cannabis, hallucinogens) can all have major effects. While there is some controversy over the relative danger of some of these substances, there is rarely any question about the danger posed by the use of heroin, unprescribed fentanyl, and some designer drugs.

The Lodge program believes that there are several major issues to think about regarding substance use by individuals suffering from NBD:

- A subset of the population, possibly more so with males, are susceptible to the potential negative effects of substance use.

- Rates of psychotic morbidity have been increasing, correlated to increased access to substances.

- There is often a relationship between use of substances, particularly marijuana, alcohol, and stimulants, and the onset of illness.

- There is an effect of substance use on recurrence of illness in individuals who have recovered or who are under treatment.

- The most recent data shows that incidence rates of Schizophrenia Spectrum Disorder are increasing with the increased use of cannabis (marijuana) in Western societies.

It is the team's view that use of substances can increase a vulnerable individual's risk of presenting with a psychotic illness or having an existing illness deteriorate further, or can lead to a recurrence of psychiatric illness after some recovery of stability has been attained. It is notable that eighty percent of Lodge patients have comorbid substance use disorders and were treated with stimulants for Attention-Deficit disorder. Therefore, the team believes strongly that both in the program and going forward, their patients must be encouraged and helped to sustain sobriety.

What are the strategies used to do this?

- **Education:** for both residents and their families. It is the repeated message of the program that doing well over an extended period of time requires 1) compliance with medication, 2) maintenance of a strong connection to treatment teams, 3) the rebuilding of social connections to family and community, 4) return to school and/or work, and 5) maintaining a generally sober lifestyle. In the experience of the team, the best outcomes have occurred when sobriety is maintained. It is understood that it is not realistic to assume that a young person who has, for example, returned to college, will never drink with their friends or that this occasional drink will be catastrophic. There exists, however, a slippery slope when it comes to substance use. The program feels that smoking marijuana constitutes a particularly dangerous path and consistently sends this message to patients. There is increasing data that supports this position. Providing this data is helpful in reducing the argument that it is "just your opinion."[7]

- **Recommendations:** If a resident is struggling to maintain sobriety post-discharge, it is recommended that they remove themselves as much as possible from triggers. This means, for example, not living close to or hanging out with friends who are using substances frequently.

- **Reminders:** The staff who remain in contact with residents post-discharge give them frequent reminders about the importance of maintaining sobriety and how substance use was problematic in their past.

- **Pharmacological support:** Sometimes cognitive and psychotherapeutic interventions are not enough, and pharmacological support is appropriate. In fact, it is the team's opinion that many patients use substances, especially marijuana, to self-medicate mood instability and some of the symptoms of psychosis. Clozapine seems to decrease impulsivity and consequently increase patients' ability to refrain from making what they know to be bad choices. This includes choices about sobriety and medication compliance. Naltrexone and naloxone, which are opiate blockers, also help to control impulsiveness, as do antiepileptic mood stabilizers like lamotrigine, which can sometimes help patients do better. In the SHH cohort, the addition of oxytocin seems to lead to even more improvement in the ability to maintain a stable and sober life.

- **Political Advocacy:** There is a general observation in addiction medicine that the craving of substances is a function of availability. Statistics on psychiatric hospital admissions, accident rates, overdose rates, emergency room visits, and suicide rates increasingly suggest that making some substances more easily available through legalization and commercialization is having a negative impact on the vulnerable young. (Details of data-based evidence can be found in the Appendix). Advocacy for further research evaluating the effects of this increased availability and education about the data that has been collected thus far is important, as is our need to increase funding for substance use disorder treatment.

PART III:
MULTIFACETED APPROACH TO
TREATMENT

THE ROLE OF EDUCATION IN LODGE TREATMENT

It might seem that understanding and recognizing the diagnosis of schizophrenia or schizoaffective illness would be fairly straightforward but understanding the true complexity of neuropsychiatric illnesses—

differentiating some of their symptoms from personality disorders and managing expectations of functioning and progress—is far more difficult than it might seem at first glance. Many families come to The Lodge having spoken to many providers and having read as much as they can in both medical and popular articles and on the internet. There is a lot of information out there, but it can be confusing, contradictory, and sometimes outdated and false. Some families have told the team that they were advised to give up and accept that their loved one would likely be institutionalized for life. Other families continue to deny the possibility of this diagnosis, afraid of the stigma and outcomes so often attached to these labels.

Our understanding of the brain and NBD is constantly evolving. From the start, the team tries to reach a better understanding of the particular case, helping patients and their families distinguish between behaviors that are attributable to a distinct personality and those that are symptoms of an underlying illness. In many ways, the long-term success of these interventions relies on patients and families understanding and accepting a complex diagnostic picture offered by the team, and its concomitant treatment protocol. This necessarily involves an openness to learning and understanding the complexities of a neuropsychiatric brain disease.

Understanding You Are Ill

Anosognosia, the denial of illness, is one of the hallmarks of NBD. When you are caught in the storm of a thought disorder, you often do not realize you are lost. In fact, you often believe that it is others who are trying to force you off course. Some patients embrace their psychotic delusions, feeling that their suffering is a sign of their special place in the universe, either as a sinner or a divinity. Others feel the world is against them, and that, too, makes them special. The team's first educational task is to convince their patients, and their families, if necessary, that they are struggling to function, and that this struggle is an illness negatively impacting their lives. For this approach to work, the team must understand a patient's individual story, which may shed light on their particular parable of suffering and isolation. This process takes time and trust. A patient has to be on medication long enough for the acuteness of their thought disorder to diminish, giving more rational thinking and belief in their doctor's perspective time to take hold.

Sometimes, especially when patients are going through extensive medical evaluations or the worst of side effects, they are insistent that the program is not what they need. It is at these moments that families often need the help of the team to tolerate their loved one's communication of discomfort and desire to leave. As a society, we have learned to accept discomfort as a necessary evil in relation to the treatment of physical illnesses like cancer and diabetes. Understanding this necessity in relation to NBD is less commonplace but just as critical. Educating both patients and their families about the biological and chemical aspects of NBD helps build this understanding.

Again, trust is central to this equation. The process of emerging from disordered thinking takes a great deal of effort from all involved. It takes time and is exponentially helped by immersion in a treatment milieu where experience and feedback occur throughout the day and sometimes in unexpected ways. To go back to our metaphor, in order to weather the storms during a voyage you need to have faith in the crew's knowledge and ability, a willingness to follow their instructions, and a developing connection to the vessel on which you sail. What happens if a loved one, despite all interventions, continues to deny that they are ill? This is an important issue to which we turn our attention in more detail in Chapter Seven.

ACCEPTING THE DIAGNOSIS OF NEUROPSYCHIATRIC BRAIN DISEASE

Once you have accepted that you or your loved one has any illness at all, you need to accept that your NBD is not attributable to something that feels less stigmatizing. With severe neuropsychiatric illness, there are often comorbidities like obsessive compulsive or borderline personality disorders, or years of substance use, which seem less frightening as diagnoses than NBD and can be used to explain away bizarre behavior. Substance use, for example, can induce transient or even long-lasting behavioral changes that are indistinguishable from major neuropsychiatric disorders. Cannabis, alcohol, opiates, and stimulants change brain chemistry and physiology. Substances can also exacerbate disorders or modify their presentation and course.

Some patients have not fit in with their peers since childhood, but others have shown early talents that make current behavior feel like it could be just a temporary derailment. Until recently, schizophrenia spectrum illnesses have been approached almost entirely as degenerative diseases, forever preventing a person from leading a life rich in community and purpose. Accepting a diagnosis of schizophrenia or schizoaffective disorder often feels like a threat to any hope of future recovery. So, it is entirely understandable that families and patients would shy away from such a diagnosis.

Living at The Lodge, residents are surrounded by peers who are at various stages of their voyage, and they are able to see parts of their own lives and struggles in those around them. There is no pretense to be "normal," and over time, residents will see peers take medication, discuss their symptoms and challenges, establish meaningful lives outside of the program, and help and support one another. This is an important part of the immersive education of The Lodge experience, complemented by the team's frequent reminders that change takes time and that the future can, in fact, be better. In a multitude of ways, residents and their families are shown repeatedly that living with NBD is not a life sentence without any hope of parole. Instead, with stabilization from acute symptoms and adherence to a treatment protocol (including medication), there is the promise of a life of agency and meaning.

REPLACING SHAME WITH OPTIMISTIC UNDERSTANDING

Education at The Lodge is sensitive to the fact that the diagnosis of NBD is also often bound to a sense of shame and failure, cultural constants, both for patients and their families. Sadly, families, particularly mothers, are still blamed too often for their loved one's illness and sometimes hold themselves accountable. While not always as overt a finger-pointing as the "schizophrenogenic mother" label of the 1950s–70s, laying responsibility for a loved one's mental decompensation on their families is still too frequent an occurrence. It is also true that it is easier to stigmatize an illness that you cannot see. Unlike a tumor or a high white blood cell count, that are visible signs of underlying physical illness, neuropsychiatric brain disease has no visible physical markers and associated behaviors are easy to misinterpret as within someone's control.

It is important to team members that education at The Lodge does not result in a sense of humiliation but instead that it replace negative, demoralizing beliefs with less judgmental, and more optimistic understanding. This occurs in a myriad of ways, ranging from education about the genetic vulnerability underlying brain disease and the neurobiology of severe brain dysfunction to the effects of stress, sociocultural issues, and substance use on vulnerable biological systems. Reducing experiences of guilt and replacing them with more pragmatic, useful frameworks is one of the team's missions.

It Is Easier to Learn When It Feels Like a Collaborative Experience

Collaboration at The Lodge occurs at every level of interaction, and staff talk openly about how much they learn from each other, as well as what they try to impart to patients and their families, and what patients and their families can impart to them. Conversations about cases happen informally in hallways and offices, and formally once a week in Rounds, a meeting attended by all the team. There, each patient's history is presented, and particularly difficult cases are discussed at length. Rounds are filled with discussions of medical conditions that may cause or mimic psychiatric symptoms, calls to consultants to weigh in on difficult cases, differentiation of behaviors from symptoms (for example, the fact that paranoia may look like rudeness and anger), relaying of historical information that may shed additional perspective on different conditions, and the inclusion of feedback from any staff who interact with patients, including those who are not tasked with direct patient care.

"You need fuel in order to be able to do this," says one team member, and Dr. Marotta speaks frequently of the importance of team morale in doing this work. Collaborative communication and a sense that you are always learning are part of what feeds that morale. Patients and their families need to feel they are part of the dialogue as well. Identifying with and being able to appreciate the positive changes you see in others is transformative. Family meetings occur weekly, and families always have access to the team. Some families and patients will need frequent contact to build trust and feel heard. Others will need to be pursued. In every case, however, the mission of the team is to work collaboratively with everyone involved. With this collaboration, over time, families often change their stance toward illness, becoming more accepting and understanding of the process. Serious bonds are often forged between patients, their families, and staff members, going far beyond pleasantries and holiday cards. Increasing a family's confidence in the process has a ripple effect. As they become more connected and trusting, their ability and interest in helping other families increases enormously.

PACE AND SCOPE OF TREATMENT IN THE LODGE

There is a paradigm for treatment at The Lodge: begin with what a resident can handle. Residents have often visited The Lodge while at the end of their stay in the ACU, so that the new environment is not entirely foreign. Sometimes, in the early stages of their stay, like Sidney who listened to inner voices and air-boxed with hallucinatory demons, residents can barely tolerate any interpersonal interaction at all. The goal of community living—working, eating, and hanging out—is never forced. A staff member might just sit on the floor with a resident or might go to their room to have a three-minute chat. Each resident is assigned a primary psychiatrist, who they have often already met during their ACU stay. They are also assigned a primary therapist social worker, but residents interact with all the staff, and if they bond with one staff member above all others, that person can become the point of contact and feedback, helping the resident to navigate through the treatment process. The fluidity of patient symptoms, personality, and the milieu of The Lodge requires a staff that is not rigid in its response. There are rules and procedures, but there are also overall objectives that must be kept in mind. The Lodge staff must be well-trained, confident, and supported so that they can be flexible when the situation requires.

Initially, the team tries to maintain some skepticism about what they are told in the paperwork that accompanies their patients. "We try to maintain a sense of wonder and excitement about discovering the underlying psychophysiological aspects of a case," says Dr. Marotta, "always hopeful that our explorations will lead to a reconceptualization of someone's particular struggle and that this will lead to a therapeutic breakthrough."

The philosophy of The Lodge program is that there are many important layers to the recovery journey, and there are many ways in which to get someone engaged in the process. Consequently, treatment in The Lodge program takes place in a variety of ways, and most importantly, relies on a continual "read" of each patient's interpersonal reactivity. During their stay, a resident will be evaluated, and their needs addressed in an individualized manner. The following is a list of some of The Lodge treatment modalities through which this will occur:

- individual therapy

- group therapy

- cognitive remediation

- active daily living skills

- exercise

- having a calm environment in which to heal

- community living.

While formal individual sessions in staff offices are scheduled a couple times a week, informal meetings between residents and their therapists happen frequently as staff members check in on their patients, often daily, or go to meetings in and out of The Lodge building. Group therapy of some kind takes place daily, addressing a large variety of interpersonal and daily living skills, and time for exercise, either at the gym or on the grounds, is built into the schedule twice a day. This belief in the important role that exercise, and a serene environment, can play in healing is reminiscent of the founding vision of Silver Hill Hospital. Residents and their families agree. Living in "a loving environment that allows all patients to find rest in a space away from traumatic energy and environmental triggers is healing," says an alum.

Practicing daily living skills is also essential to building a life that has agency. When residents enter The Lodge program, they are often so psychotic that their ability to focus on simple tasks of self-care or household chores is minimal or nonexistent. As medication takes effect and residents become more self-aware, their ability to perform and participate in these skills of daily living improves. Structuring time for household chores in the schedule is a way of drawing attention to both the importance of individual responsibility and community membership. SHH hosts other support group meetings in the evening, which Lodge residents are welcome to attend, but most residents are too early in their recovery process to focus on activities beyond The Lodge community.

Information from all these elements of a resident's daily routine is shared and integrated into the evolving treatment plan. Weekly Rounds, collaborative discussions, and spontaneous informal gatherings in staff members' offices are the norm. Nor are all discussions and decisions specific to individual cases. Decisions regarding community functioning are also key to the success of the program, and community structure can change depending on the profile of current patients. A decision to hold formal community meetings may work with one group of residents, for example, but some months later may not be possible with another group. The ability to assess and adapt is critical when you are dealing with a wide diversity of symptoms and personalities. Each time a new patient is admitted to The Lodge program, the team understands that the dynamics of the community will be affected and must be reevaluated.

FLEXIBILITY AND CREATIVITY OF APPROACH

Flexibility and creativity in therapeutic work require a sensitivity to the needs of your patients, a willingness to part from more rigid ideology, and the confidence and support necessary to act. At The Lodge, all staff are encouraged to be flexible and get creative, and routines are adaptable. For example, morning blood work can be done later if a resident is unable to rise early. This sounds insignificant but it is not. Remember, many members of The Lodge program are taking clozapine, which can be quite sedating, especially in the beginning. Allowing them to get their blood work later both validates their experience and makes accomplishing this task much easier.

Each resident has a primary therapist but interacts with most of the team members during their stay, which helps the process of community integration and allows the team to get feedback about each patient from different staff members. Residential counselors help residents to transition to The Lodge in whatever ways they can. This can take place in their room, in the common room, helping them to get exercise or play a game if they ask. As residents become clearer in their thinking, they may begin to go to their therapist's office for their sessions and to attend different group therapies. They may also begin going to the gym to exercise or go to the hospital cafe with a staff member for lunch. The ability to widen the arc of their activity on the SHH campus is one sign that a resident is getting better.

Let's take a moment to see an example of creative therapeutics at work in The Lodge program.

The Cooking Group: a Peephole into the Ship's Galley

The cooking group, run by social workers Jackie Ordoñez, LCSW, and Kate Welzel, LCSW, is a wonderful example of how all the elements of The Lodge voyage come together to support change. Flexibility of approach, therapeutic attention to communication and interpersonal issues, medication, time, and patience all contribute to the success of this group experience. Let's look at this working group more closely.

Jackie tells us that she raised the idea of beginning a cooking group at The Lodge based on her memory of a program at a different house where the RCs cooked with the residents. Communal cooking no longer exists in that house, but the idea of residents working together to prepare a meal intrigued her, and with the support of the team, she began to plan a cooking group for The Lodge residents. She needed to think through how they could involve up to fourteen acutely ill patients in preparing a full meal while keeping everyone safe, especially since using a knife is necessary in meal preparation.

Before the initial group meeting, Jackie and Kate, her co-leader, assigned each of the patients a task appropriate to their current level of functioning, and wrote it on a large chart hung up on the two Lodge refrigerators. "Here are your jobs," they told the residents when they arrived for group. Residents and their jobs were color-coded. "Check your color and find your job." Laughing, Jackie says, "It was a total fail!" Taking initiative was difficult for many residents, and some didn't know how to do the simplest of tasks, like boiling pasta. Back to the drawing board.

It was clear that self-guided activities would not work. Maybe telling residents their assignments individually, ahead of time, was the path. While better, this plan still didn't work well enough. Residents' functioning can be very fluid, especially in the early stages of their treatment. What became clear was that even if a resident had had a good day the day before, or even a good period forty-five minutes before the group, that did not guarantee they would be functioning well when the group began. The clinical pathway had been defined: adapting to the needs of each resident in the moment was imperative. Deciding who could use a knife or who needed more space and should only wash dishes had to wait until the group started.

Now, in the current group structure, tasks are assigned only when group begins and group members can be assessed. Meal planning decisions are never made too far in advance either. Patients who cannot tolerate interaction in any form do not attend the group, but limited capacity for interaction does not prohibit group participation. If a resident needs to rock in the corner, they are given the space, and their participation may involve only taking out an ingredient or washing one dish. By the time they leave the program, however, most residents have learned quite a lot in the cooking group, and kitchen skills are only one treatment variable among many.

Cooking group is, in its own way, a microcosm of life. What is learned and practiced are a set of skills that help residents live life with agency. Throughout the group, Jackie and Kate model behavior and how to talk to one another, a critical skill for people whose sense of empathic connection to others has been weakened or lost. There is constant verbal and nonverbal communication within the group, and Jackie and Kate help residents to process this and respond appropriately. Working in a kitchen setting also requires residents to learn respect for each other's personal space, how to share, how to work as a team, how to prioritize tasks, and how to hang with friends and colleagues in a less formal manner. Importantly, it develops necessary life skills in a physically and emotionally safe environment. Knowing how to cook and clean up after oneself are simple but fundamental tasks. But ordering a patient to clean up is not nearly as effective as incorporating this skill as part of the process, for example, saying, "Let's make dessert and then clean up afterward." Whether a resident is living on their own, in community housing, or back with their family when they leave the hospital, the knowledge and ability to share this kind of responsibility is one piece of living a more empowered life.

As medication helps to quiet acute symptoms, a resident's increased functioning in the cooking group is a useful and sometimes early marker of their overall progress in the program. Take Ian, for example, whose changing participation in the cooking group is a beautiful illustration of his increasing psychological integration.

Ian's Story

Ian was in his late twenties when he arrived at Silver Hill Hospital. Prior to his arrival, he had completely isolated himself to a confined space in his family's home and hadn't left the home in a very long time. Upon arriving at Silver Hill, he was extremely paranoid, guarded, and delusional. Looking like a cave-dweller, with a long beard and shaggy long hair, he had significant delusions regarding his family and refused to have anything to do with them. During his early days in The Lodge program, he was often difficult to engage, though he would attend most programming offered.

In the cooking group, he was initially guarded, but as time went on his guard started to drop slowly. As medication softened some of his most acute symptoms, he began to participate more actively and appeared more at ease. He began to smile, make eye contact, engage in small talk not only with peers but also with staff running the group, and on occasion, even made a couple of jokes. He had worked in a family restaurant and so often stepped in to share with peers a more effective way of doing things or helped the staff demonstrate various cooking techniques. He still experienced paranoia and delusions related to his family and wouldn't talk to any of his therapists directly about them, but in the context of the cooking group he was able to engage in superficial conversation about his family, which was a significant marker of change.

By the end of his time in The Lodge program, he took pride in preparing meals for the house as a whole. As he completed his meal preparation he would say, "It's time to gather the family for dinner." This was a remarkable statement from someone whose early psychotic paranoia had led to complete isolation and worries that his family would harm him.

Ian moved to a step-down community for a period of a year following his time at The Lodge and continued to see both his therapist and psychiatrist from the program. Just recently, he has left this supervised housing and is living on his own, once again connected to family members. He is working while still continuing on the medication regimen started at The Lodge.

The Importance of Communication

Complexity of communication is at the heart of all therapeutic work, and clear and constant communication is essential to the work at The Lodge. It takes place on many different levels, in many ways beyond the overt denotation of words (such as pauses, facial expressions, postures, and eye contact), all which must be acknowledged and respected by the team. Here are some of its many layers at The Lodge:

- staff to patients, and patients to staff

- staff to family members, and family members to staff

- staff to staff on the same shift, and staff to staff on different shifts

- patients to patients

- staff to admissions/administration, and admissions/administration to staff

- staff to consultants, and consultants to staff

- staff to previous therapists/psychiatrists, and previous therapists/psychiatrists to staff

- staff to insurance companies, and insurance companies to staff

- staff to follow-up step-down programs or community teams, and those programs/teams to staff.

Residents can behave differently in different contexts, can both conceal and reveal, and what might be seen by one staff member may be invisible to others. Let's take Y, for example, who stays in his room without saying anything about his gastrointestinal symptoms, which are only discovered because housekeeping reports signs of illness in his bathroom. Or Z, who denies hearing voices when speaking to their doctor, but is seen by a residential counselor carrying on an animated conversation with someone who is not there as they smoke a cigarette on the back patio. W, another resident, may participate easily in activities of daily living in a seemingly normal manner but confide to one staff member that she is really God.

In all these instances, it is only through communication with each other that the team gets a full and rounded understanding of their residents' struggles. Similarly, communications with residents' families need to be shared and discussed to avoid the possibility that staff will be split in their responses and mixed messages given. When families are anxious, they may put pressure on the different members of the team. Keeping lines of communication open with each other allows the team to stay uniform in their responses and gives them greater insight into the nature of patient-family dynamics. Continued communication also helps staff to gain insight into their own and their patients' transferential responses. With seriously ill patients, eruptions triggered by family and friends can cause parallel stress within the team. Understanding and recognizing these group dynamics allows staff to process their experience and maintain the equilibrium necessary to handle stressful disruption.

The Lodge team must also interface and work smoothly with a number of other teams, both within the SHH structure and outside with other institutions and agencies. For example, clear communication is equally critical between The Lodge team and SHH Admissions, as it helps to protect the integrity of the program as well as the efficient and safe functioning of the hospital. When Admissions suggests a new patient for the program, the needs of each current resident are considered, and The Lodge team assesses whether or not they feel the new candidate will fit in.

The Admissions staff must also evaluate the physical, medical, and emotional state of a potential patient so that a potentially catastrophic problem, such as severe withdrawal from substances, is anticipated and treated. The hospital has a mission to serve but is also a business. The ongoing dialogue between The Lodge staff and Admissions sometimes reflects the tension between this dialectic. There is a lot of give and take, but The Lodge team realizes it is luckier than most. It gets enormous institutional support.

Repeated communication with insurance companies, while an ongoing challenge, is also a necessary part of the process. Team members frequently argue with insurance companies for hours trying to get more time for their patients. They also coach families on how to do the same. It is one of the ongoing frustrations to the team that these hours on the phone take away from direct patient care. In fact, the securing of finances is a major problem for the vast majority of medical institutions in our country. It is a significant factor, not only in the delivery of high quality, effective care but also in the equity of access. This is a critical issue: more patients need to be afforded the opportunity to access programs like The Lodge.

THE IMPORTANCE OF TIME AND PERSEVERANCE

The great writer Leo Tolstoy said, "The two most powerful warriors are patience and time." There is no way around it: meaningful recovery beyond the reduction of acute symptoms, for most people, takes a significant period of time. When you ask team members to name some of the most important elements contributing to their program's success, it is not surprising that time is one of the first variables they mention. "If we rely on the insurance companies for the time we need, we will be defeated. It is the families that buy us the time to do what we do. They are buying the 'War Bonds' and paying the 'taxes,' and that keeps the hospital and its program in the game!" says Dr. Marotta.

"Nobody approaches the treatment of cancer in four weeks," says Suma Srishaila, MD. "Everybody approaches cancer in one to two years, right? Nobody says, 'one cycle of treatment and figure it out on your own.' That's what we do with NBD. You have a shot in the hospital, then figure it out on your own. And that's why typical hospital stays are crazy."

The staff at The Lodge are patient. Take the example of Linda, who arrived at The Lodge scared and totally withdrawn. As RC Elaina Cardascia relates:

> The way she handled her fear, and being overwhelmed, was just to be angry and mean. She was so scared. . . . she never left her room. So we started by accommodating her, and that was step one. We would bring meals to her, we would go to her to talk, and then we started slowly bringing her out a little. Slowly, we got her to stay in the kitchen during groups, which is one room over, and then we got her to sit with her face to the group room, and then we got her to *be* in the group room, and now she's actually participating.

While acute symptoms may be decreased in a relatively shorter period, the process of rebuilding a more integrated, connected life when you struggle with NBD often requires a much more gradual approach, one that continues for months after discharge from the program. It often requires teasing apart the complexity of symptoms and then titrating changes slowly. For example, said a former team member, reminiscing about the process of teasing apart a diagnosis:

> Let's say that somebody is defensive and short. Somebody could perceive them as an asshole, right? And instead, they're paranoid. . . . they're scared. You didn't see the scared. You saw somebody that was mean or abrasive, or you want to classify it into a personality piece instead of a poor soul protecting themselves against a failing mind, you know? And many times, people would be diagnosed with personality disorders who came to us, but we saw symptoms that were a defense mechanism, not a diagnosis.

Dr. Marotta adds:

> In therapeutic circles, the label of personality disorder is often given to particularly difficult patients. It's a way of saying, "not much we can do here," but set limits and hope for the best. We believe, however, that often our patients' personality interactions are state-dependent. For example, if

they are in withdrawal from an opiate, they may appear manipulative and irritable, or in a psychotic state they may appear dismissive and paranoid. These are better seen as *pseudo*-personality disorders, thought states that may respond to concern, direction, medication, and time. Human connection is critical.

The team is acutely aware of what a gift it is that many of their patients are able to live at The Lodge for periods that far exceed a typical hospital stay. It is only with time that these layers of illness can be stripped away, and the earlier in a patient's psychotic decompensation this can be done the better. The need to reverse the disease process before it becomes fixed is considered paramount.

Extended time at The Lodge allows for:

- repeated medication trials, medication titration, and adjustment

- reduction of acute (positive) symptoms

- attention to underlying emotional (negative) symptoms and personality issues

- building active daily living skills

- rebuilding trust with others

- reconnecting with outside communities

- developing healthier nutrition and lifestyle habits

- developing the tolerance and coping mechanisms to deal with stress

- internalizing an acceptance of the fact that NBD is a chronic illness

DEALING WITH TURBULENCE

"First, do no harm" has been a central tenet of medicine since ancient times, but when working with resistant NBD, there is always a tension between acting with caution and taking the necessary risks to get your patient well. The team is always trying to predict where failure and disruption might occur and to take warranted precautions, but with NBD there are many variables which are difficult to predict and even harder to control. It is impossible to get it right all the time. Understanding that adjustment is part of the process helps patients and their families better tolerate moments when things don't seem to be working well in the treatment process.

Part of the skill of a captain and crew is to navigate the turbulence when the waters get rough. With NBD, turbulence can occur for many reasons. For example:

- A resident's behavior at The Lodge can become too disruptive or unsafe (medication is not working or outside stressors cause an eruption).

- A resident's blood work may indicate a dangerous response to medication.

- A resident (or their family) may become impatient while medication trials are underway and push for premature action.

- A resident may become physically ill.

- A new roommate or resident at The Lodge may be disruptive or difficult to handle, disturbing what may have felt like a safe and comfortable therapeutic milieu (the staff will always attempt to address this immediately and make necessary changes or accommodations to try to regain a calm milieu).

- A world event or major personal event (e.g., a death in the family) may cause significant trauma that interrupts a treatment regimen that has been effective.

- A resident may not disclose psychotic or depressive ideation (psychotic paranoia facilitates keeping secrets) and then behave in a surprising manner.

- A resident's family may act intrusively and create stress for the patient and/or staff.

- Staff has to spend hours arguing with insurance companies that are denying what the team considers necessary treatment.

- A discharged resident may not continue to take their medication, leading to relapse of symptoms, exploitation by others, overdose, suicide, or violent behavior.

- A staff member may need coverage or support during a personal emergency.

Responding to turbulence requires the experience to assess the situation, the ability to recognize both individual and group dynamics, and the skills and resources to actualize the appropriate response. Listening to one another is key. Dr. Marotta's door is always open to staff who want to vent or talk something over, and it is not unusual to find staff hanging with each other in someone's office, talking over a problem or reviewing a difficult day. Dr. Marotta also checks in regularly with staff he doesn't often see, like team members on the night shift. They know that he is available night or day. Individual support, as well as group dynamics, get his attention because the morale of the team is his biggest priority after patient care. It is important to understand that resilience and persistence are essential factors in the NBD journey. It is also important to understand that both families and professionals need support to sustain their resourceful functioning.

PUTTING IT ALL TOGETHER

Many of you know how complex the voyage is through the storm of acute NBD. There are many ways to get capsized or driven off course. The Lodge program was developed from years of experience navigating these pitfalls and developing an approach that helps a patient's journey to stability be as smooth and successful as possible. As with most travel, not everything is predictable. Getting from one stop to the next can require detours and changes of plans. The Lodge treatment team has developed strategies that respond flexibly to the needs of their patients while maintaining a commitment to the underlying tenets of the program.

Are you unable to access The Lodge program itself? The information contained in this chapter is still useful as a guide to pursuing potential treatment resources. Understanding how The Lodge program differs from "standard" acute care treatment can help you in your evaluation of other programs. We recognize that the reality of what is available to your loved one at any one point in time may be

Continued ➤

limited, and that other effective treatment facilities won't necessarily model every aspect of The Lodge. But knowing what to look for can guide your search when you have options. Here are the key ideas that form the foundation of The Lodge treatment approach.

KEY IDEAS FOR CHAPTER FIVE: THE LODGE VOYAGE

FOUNDATIONAL COMPONENTS

- **Trust**: The gift of time in a long-term residential program allows for the development of the essential trusting relationship between patients, families, and the treatment team.

- **Flexibility and creativity of approach**: Weekly Rounds, collaborative discussions, and spontaneous informal gatherings in staff members' offices are the norm. These collaborations constantly inform the multifaceted treatment plan for each patient.

- **Education**: Teaching about the underlying causes of NBD helps to replace shame with optimistic understanding.

- **Communication**: Clear and constant communication between staff, patients, families, and all treatment providers within and outside the program is necessary.

- **Time and patience:** Time and patience are necessary to distinguish physical and personality variables from psychotic processes, to effect medication trials, and to allow both staff and peer modeling of behavior to take effect.

AREAS OF FOCUS WITHIN THE LODGE PROGRAM

- **Medication management and compliance**: You need a program with the staff, support, and time to allow for suc-

Continued ➤

cessful medication trials, titrations, and changes to each particular patient's medication regimen.

- **Clozapine**: This atypical antipsychotic has been proven to have a transformational effect on those with NBD, and a program like this provides all the necessary support, with time to allow it to be successfully onboarded.

- **Oxytocin**: This neuropeptide has been extraordinarily powerful in helping patients with NBD (usually on clozapine) to connect and relate to others when their more acute positive symptoms (e.g., delusions, hallucinations, disordered thinking) have been reduced.

- **Sobriety**

- **Building activities of daily living,** healthy habits, and connection to peers

- **Reconnecting a patient to family**

- **Building a patient's community** and their ability to form relationships

- **Helping a patient develop a sense of personal agency** so that they can engage in school, work, and self-care

OXYTOCIN
—An Alum's Story

Before I started taking oxytocin, I remember being scared of other people.

This was true for everyone except for the few people I was closest with—my parents, and a few close friends.

For the rest—strangers and acquaintances (the latter category I applied to people who could have been called "friends"—that's how anxious and distrustful I was of others)—I felt a kind of pressure, almost physical, long before I even tried to speak with them.

For example: sometimes I would be invited as part of a group to have dinner at a nearby restaurant. I would drive myself there, park my car, and sit quietly by myself, already thinking at a rapid-fire pace, "I shouldn't be here. No one wants me to be here. If there are already people sitting inside, they are likely talking about how annoyed they are that I'll be joining them—that I shouldn't have been invited, that I embarrass myself whenever I try to speak." And then, I'd see a handful of people from our group standing together outside the restaurant, chatting among themselves.

That's when it would start. "Have they noticed I'm here?" I'd think to myself, looking across the parking lot, already embarrassed at myself for trying to see if they were aware that I'd arrived. To me, that would be the worst outcome: they'd see me, sitting in my car, alone, and take that as yet another example of me being socially awkward to the point of being a public embarrassment.

I use this word a lot, "embarrassment," because that's exactly what my problem was at the time. I was at that point stable enough medically that my emotions didn't fluctuate sharply between extremes. However, while I was stable, I wasn't happy—I was dissatisfied with myself, because I still had a painful fear of being around other people, when I desperately wanted to be. I felt the gap between the social relationships I wanted to build and my ability to be social. Thus, when I would try to be social, I felt like I was in a constant state of self-embarrassment—which I would "feel" (but really imagined) by assuming the thoughts running in everyone else's minds, which invariably were disparaging toward myself.

I would start imagining these thoughts once any person looked at

Continued ➤

me. Even if, for example, I was halfway across a dimly lit parking lot, walking toward them but out of earshot, I would imagine their thoughts. They would start quickly, and move quickly, like my own. They would jump from tangent to tangent but would all be centered on me—this embarrassment who was nothing more than a social parasite, making everyone around myself irritated and uncomfortable.

Unsurprisingly, this would get worse when I'd be close enough to start a conversation with them. Back then, trying to start a conversation with someone was agonizing. I wanted, really wanted, to talk casually with these people about something, anything—but I didn't know where to start.

That's when I'd get angry at myself. I'd think, "Well, what the hell am I supposed to say now? Look at them, they're all staring at me, no, they're glaring, they're already pissed off that I decided to show up tonight. And now it's been how many seconds since I intruded on their conversation? They hate me. They all hate me. I should leave. But that would be even worse. If I turned around and left without saying a word, that would be the ultimate display of me being completely socially incompetent. And then I'd have no chance, none, of ever having some sort of acquaintance with them."

This mix of thoughts, blending my irritation at myself with the imagined internal narratives of the people around me, came with something I mentioned before—a pressure of sorts. It's hard to describe—but I remember feeling it throughout my body, like a weight pressing down on me, feeling heaviest in my head. It made it twice as difficult to look people directly in the eye, which I already struggled with given my lack of self-confidence.

I also felt jittery—I'd suddenly feel physically energetic (something which was otherwise unusual for me, as I more often felt lethargic in my day-to-day life). This also increased my difficulty in making eye contact or maintaining it for more than a few seconds before quickly looking elsewhere out of shame.

Finally, the combination of these physical sensations and my thought patterns distorted my sense of time when I was around other people. Sometimes, I'd become aware of my spike in energy and feel as if everyone else around me was talking more slowly, or that at least my perceptions were sped-up. Other times, when I focused on trying to start a

Continued ➤

conversation, I'd feel like I was the one moving slower than everyone else, mainly because I was jumping into multiple people's heads at once, all getting irritated at me for being too slow to speak or respond appropriately to their remarks.

In retrospect, all of this meant that while I was imagining these disparaging thoughts directed at myself, I was unable to hear what these people were in fact talking about. I'd only pick up on a word or two in a brief moment of calming myself down, and then panic again, realizing I hadn't been paying attention, which would create another set of problems trying to join in. Additionally, on a rare occasion when I challenged myself to enter into a conversation, I would speak clumsily, slurring a syllable or needing to restart what I was saying altogether. And that would seriously discourage me from ever trying to speak to the people in question again.

This was what it was like for me to be in social situations before I took oxytocin. When I started taking it, the changes I felt weren't instantaneous. It took time—both my body getting used to the medication itself and continued therapy to work through my own thoughts. But within the first year of taking it, I remember a few changes.

Both the physical sensations—the pressure and jitters—and my habit of jumping into other people's heads started fading away. They became less a constant once people saw me, and more based on the situation. If I was walking toward a crowd, similar to the example I mentioned earlier, they'd only start if there were people I had identified (for one reason or another) as people I'd realistically like to spend my time with. It wasn't that anyone and everyone thought I was an embarrassment and an irritant—it was more about me being self-conscious of my still-fledgling interpersonal skills with people I wanted to build relationships with.

Also, if I was in a large group and was asked or prompted to speak, I would feel the pressure and jitters—though more mild than before—and wouldn't spend time automatically imagining other people's thoughts. I was able to speak, if only a sentence or two, and still stumbling on a word here and there.

When I'd talk about these moments anecdotally in therapy, I began to realize with my therapist that I was making progress. I, literally for the first time in my life, was getting better at talking to other people.

This encouraged me to keep trying, even though it scared me. It went a long way for me that, in therapy, I had a safe space to talk about

Continued ➤

these little "victories" of mine—moments that were a huge deal to me but would seem minuscule and silly to most anyone else.

As my therapist pointed out to me over time, I was catching up to learning the social skills most people pick up naturally when they're younger. That thought made me bitter sometimes (and it still does), as I'd become resentful that I had to make up for so much lost time, through no fault of my own. But on the flip side, I was making progress. I had the means to make progress. Before I started taking oxytocin, I didn't have that. I was paralyzed and had no way to move forward. But now, I did.

After that, the next several years brought many changes for me, internally and externally. Internally, I started making big changes to how I thought about myself and other people. These changes came through the conversations I'd have in therapy—but were absolutely made possible by those initial changes I mentioned feeling when I started taking oxytocin. And, as taking oxytocin became normal for me, an afterthought in my daily life, that's when I was able to do the hard work on myself.

My therapist once pointed out to me that I was putting other people on a pedestal compared to myself. And I'd reply, "Well, of course I am, because. . . ." and I'd list things I hated about myself. But I've since been able to see myself in a more positive light. I started caring less what other people thought about me. I started forgiving myself more easily when I spoke awkwardly during a conversation. I generally put less blame on myself than before—and I allowed myself to get angry, to feel justified in my own actions. I wasn't, by default, in the wrong in all situations.

Finally, when I did "mess up" in a social situation, I was more readily able to let it go. Sometimes that would take some breathing, often a bit of self-care to calm down, but it wouldn't overwhelm my thoughts for the rest of the day or evening—I could move on.

It's been roughly seven years since I started taking oxytocin. The person I am today is completely different from who I was, and my life is extraordinary: I've accomplished things, inside and out, my old self would think impossible.

Some of these impossible things include being able to strike up a conversation, being able to look other people in the eye, being able to walk in a crowded place without imagining everyone thinking negatively about me. I can walk down a street thinking about what groceries I need to buy or what time I need to set my morning alarm for, rather than berating

Continued ➤

myself for a social faux pas three days ago that should keep me from ever leaving my apartment again.

Most of all, I see myself as someone who has a right to live in this world—a world where most people learned in childhood and adolescence the social skills I've been working to develop since my mid-twenties.

I still worry sometimes what other people think of me during a conversation and, in moments of stress, may jump into the other person's head and imagine their negativity toward me. But I can shut that down quickly, because I recognize it as my own behavior and not reality—and, even if they think that way about me, that's okay. It doesn't mean I have to.

If anything, what I struggle with today is that resentment of time lost for developing my social skills. Today, I'll let myself feel that anger, let myself recognize that it is unfair, that I didn't do anything to deserve my diagnosis or circumstances—but then I remind myself that being bitter won't change that reality, that I should make the most of the time I have, and that, most importantly, I have the means to *do so*.

Chapter 6

CHARTING THE COURSE

"The pessimist complains about the wind, the optimist hopes it will turn, the realist adjusts the sails."

—*William Arthur Ward*

This chapter is a peephole into the enormous and detailed work that is required when developing a medication plan that goes beyond quieting the positive symptoms of persistent psychosis to facilitating the realization of a purposeful life. There is skill and experience involved in developing a successful treatment of NBD but no magic. Each time a medication is changed, the staff, patients, and family must wait to see its effect. There is no rushing this process, and we thought it illuminating to show you what individualized, time-consuming, and detail-oriented treatment actually looks like.

We have documented different types of illness presentations to provide a glimpse into the complexity involved in each individual case. The young men and women whose journey has led them to Silver Hill Hospital and The Lodge program have usually had psychotic decompensations that have taken place over a long period of time, with multiple hospitalizations or years of dysfunction despite treatment, and they have not responded well to conventional interventions. Ongoing treatment of NBD involves a complex dance, as the treatment team monitors an individual's stability and continuously responds to their changing life situations, which prompts medication and psychotherapeutic adjustments. It should be noted that in order to do this work, the team needs the time and stability that these patients' families can offer them by agreeing to an extended stay at The Lodge. It is this partnership which allows the work in the program to continue to maximize potential, and in many cases, to continue past discharge into a therapeutic relationship which can support good life choices. In some cases, life goals are achieved that were previously thought unattainable. To do this work takes attention to detail that never stops. It is a heroic and never-ceasing collaboration between patients, families, and their doctors.

Los Tres Amigos

Jonathan, William, and Charlie, three young adult men who represent a frequent category of patients at The Lodge, get admitted to SHH at the same time, grossly psychotic, having undergone repeatedly unsuccessful conventional antipsychotic treatment. They are all in their early twenties; all three had used substances; two had been too disorganized to graduate college; all have normal MRIs, EEGs, and blood work; and all have undergone psychological testing which shows a schizophrenic profile. Despite many similarities, however, their responses to some of the same medication trials are not always the same. They are a good example of how patients who carry a similar diagnosis and superficial history are not alike and deserve careful observation and individualized treatment planning.

At SHH, they are all placed on **clozapine (Clozaril)** with an initially good response.

Jonathan

Jonathan stays at The Lodge for three months.

- He remains so tired on clozapine that he cannot function and is moved to **quetiapine (Seroquel)** instead. A slow reduction of his acute hallucinations and delusions is observed.

- **Oxytocin** is added to address continued emotional disconnectedness and withdrawal. It helps, but the team feels things could be even better.

- **Armodafinil (Nuvigil)** is added to increase Jonathan's attentiveness. It does not help and is removed from the regimen.

- **Lamotrigine (Lamictal)** is added to address depression, especially bipolar variants. It also protects against the possible risk of seizure.

- **Lithium** is added to address mood instability.

- **Sertraline (Zoloft)** is added to address his residual depression and obsessiveness.

Jonathan is **discharged to** his family's home, where he lives for a year. He continues to be followed by Dr. Marotta and members of the team and remains friends with Charlie and William.

- During the Covid epidemic, he takes some classes.

- He begins doing volunteer work.

- He takes advanced graduate courses and eventually begins a degree program.

- He becomes entrepreneurial.

Post-discharge management: Jonathan has a great deal of energy and very high intelligence. He is very engaging, social, and playful, but also quite self-assured. This makes giving him advice more difficult since he likes to do things his way, including altering his medications as he sees fit. Maintaining an alliance is particularly important in the service of helping him see a different perspective and helping him weather moments when his decision to reduce medication is destabilizing. His activities make his management challenging, as does his willingness to take risks. Continued check-ins by Dr. Marotta are critical to sustaining a relationship of this type, with its various ups and downs.

CHARLIE

Charlie stays at The Lodge for six and a half months.

- On **clozapine**, he shows a reduction of acute hallucinations and delusions. However, he still shows some thought disorder, preoccupations, and strange thinking.

- **Haloperidol (Haldol)** is added to address these residual positive symptoms.

- **Oxytocin** is added to address his continuing signs of emotional disconnectedness.

- **Armodafinil (Nuvigil)** is added to increase attentiveness.

Charlie is **discharged to** a residential program in the city.

- He takes classes remotely during the Covid epidemic.

- Over the next year and a half, he accelerates his coursework and then transfers to a highly competitive university, taking a heavy load of courses. He is taken off haloperidol because he is doing well, and the fewer medications needed, the better.

Post-discharge management: Charlie can get paranoid and distressed. When that happens, occasionally a little bit of haloperidol is added to his regime. He is careful, self-monitors, and anticipates something going wrong. He wants to be stable and sees sobriety as critical to his health. He keeps in close contact with Dr. Marotta and remains friends with Jonathan and William. Continuing to improve, month after month, he takes great joy in his coursework and mastering new knowledge. He has become close with his family after many years of disconnection and has also developed a small social life off-campus.

William

William stays at The Lodge for four months.

- On **clozapine**, he shows a reduction of acute hallucinations and delusions.

- **Oxytocin** is added to address the remaining symptoms of emotional disconnectedness.

- **Armodafinil (Nuvigil)** is added to increase attentiveness.

- William is **discharged to** a residential program in the city.

- He takes some courses remotely during the Covid epidemic.

- He transfers to an in-person college as he had been unable to complete many credits in his previous schooling.

- He accelerates the amount of coursework to a full load.

- He starts a part-time job.

Post-discharge management: William is followed by Dr. Marotta. He can feel very sedated from the clozapine, so around school exam time his clozapine doses are decreased. When study demands decrease, his dose is increased again in order to prevent breakthrough psychosis, and he responds well to Dr. Marotta's reminders that medication compliance is important and substance use is a poor choice. He graduates with honors from college and is now working full-time. He plans to go to graduate school. He has some friends but still struggles with his desire to have a more active social life.

ZEBRAS AMONG THE HORSES

Lawrence, Anna, Josh, and Leslie are good examples of how important a good evaluation is to the development of a successful treatment plan for individuals with NBD. All four come to SHH carrying the diagnosis of schizophrenia, but close assessment leads the team to conclude that an overlooked aspect of their illness is that they exhibit behaviors that are also seen in patients with certain forms of epilepsy. Why is this important? Because if this contributing factor is overlooked, their vulnerability to experiencing psychotic symptoms will never be fully treated.

Historically, antiseizure medications were added to antipsychotic medications to improve their effectiveness, and this sometimes works. There has also been a history of literature in neurology describing the relationship of seizures to psychotic states. Overt seizures, with concomitant changes in EEG and even sometimes findings on brain imaging, are often accompanied by changes in behavior. There are cases, especially with the abnormality of brain tissues causing a seizure in the temporal or frontal lobes, that also, over time, present as a psychotic illness. This psychosis, which can look very much like schizophrenia or bipolar illness, is due to the malfunctioning brain tissue, not the seizure itself. If the same regions of the brain that are affected by conventional schizophrenia are in the area of epileptic induction (called the focus), then it is not so strange that major disruptions of behaviors, perception, cognition, and social relatedness can also be found. It is also important to note that alcohol and other substances that can be abused can lower the seizure threshold.

Up until this point in their lives, Lawrence, Josh, Anna, and Leslie have been dysfunctional, with substance use, sexual acting out, and erratic behavior forming part of their different histories. Both women are possible victims of sexual trauma, based on symptoms. All of them have acted so strangely at times that they were thought to be intoxicated. Anna has spent years in and out of hospitals and has been unsuccessfully treated with multiple antipsychotics as well as ECT (which may have exacerbated her symptoms). All of them have been in and out of confusional states. They all mention that certain substances, i.e., benzodiazepines, help them deal with symptoms, but previous doctors have felt this was just a reflection of addiction to substance use.

- Lawrence and Josh both say alcohol and benzodiazepines help them. When Josh is confused, people think he has been drinking or using drugs.

- Anna says diazepam (Valium) helps her. She is religiously preoccupied, writes a great deal, and paints incessantly.

- Leslie uses many substances and says clonazepam (Klonopin) stops her "tripping," those states of dissociation and confusion.

As a result of extensive evaluation and consultations, the team comes to believe that the four patients' desire to use alcohol, Klonopin, Valium, and other benzodiazepines has been not just addictive behavior but an attempt to self-medicate. In each of the cases, past treatment has interpreted disorganized, dissociation states as the result of substance use, but The Lodge team believes this is not entirely accurate. Consequently, in some cases benzodiazepines have been reintroduced in appropriate measures to augment the effects of other medication.

Lawrence

Lawrence stays at The Lodge for almost three months.

- He is placed on **clozapine**, and it appears helpful, but he is then **taken off clozapine** on the advice of a consulting cardiologist due to blood work showing that one cardiac enzyme is elevated.

- He is placed on high-dose **quetiapine (Seroquel)**.

- Lawrence is sent for a consultation with a senior epilepsy specialist, based on positive results on a seizure checklist.

- **Divalproex (Depakote)** is added to treat a presumptive diagnosis of partial complex seizures.

- **Amphetamine/dextroamphetamine (Adderall)** is added to help him with concentration and focus.

- **Propranolol (Inderal)** is added to address chronic autonomic instability and anxiety.

- **Lorazepam (Ativan)** is added to suppress Lawrence's residual anxiety and add seizure control.

- **Oxytocin** is added to address issues of social anxiety.

Lawrence is **discharged to** a residential program in a city.

- He goes to school. His discharge note mentions his intelligence, the clarity of his thinking, and his ability for abstract thought. He has always been a good writer, and now he is able to use his obsessive energy in his studies.

- He applies to graduate school and completes an intensive program. He is now working as a full-time professional, is in a relationship, and maintains sobriety.

Post-discharge management: Lawrence is followed by Dr. Marotta.

Anna

Anna stays at The Lodge for four months.

- She is placed on **clozapine**, which helps to reduce acute positive symptoms.

- She is sent for a consultation with a senior epilepsy specialist, based on positive results on a seizure checklist, as well as her religious preoccupation and incessant painting, which are all signs suggestive of temporal lobe seizures.

- **Lamotrigine (Lamictal)** is added to address Anna's mood instability and seizure risk.

- **Gabapentin (Neurontin)** is added to address her anxiety and seizure risk.

- **Oxytocin** is added to address issues of social disconnectedness.

- Anna continues to paint. As time goes on, her paintings change from cluttered layers of black and red paint to more coherent, representational work.

Anna is **discharged to** a long-term residential program. The team wishes she had stayed longer, as they feel they could have attained an even better outcome. The program she is in now does not mandate sobriety. The team feels this is an error.

Post-discharge management: The Lodge team works with her program to arrange treatment with another psychiatry team. They have taken over her care.

Josh

Josh stays at The Lodge for four months.

- He is placed on **clozapine**, which reduces his acute positive symptoms.

- He is sent for a consultation with a senior epilepsy specialist, based on a careful review of past history, which mentions a long-ago neurology consult that suggested seizure activity but which has not been considered significant by previous treatment teams.

- **Lamotrigine (Lamictal)** is added to address Josh's mood instability and seizure risk.

- **Depakote** is added to treat seizure risk.

- **Gabapentin (Neurontin)** is added to address anxiety and seizure risk.

- **Clonazepam (Klonopin)** is added to address seizure risk and anxiety.

- **Oxytocin** is added to address his social anxiety and emotional withdrawal.

Josh is **discharged to** live with his family.

- He gets a car and begins to live a normal life after years of being incapacitated by his illness.

- He takes up his art again. He is a talented artist, and his family reports he has returned to a high level of productivity not seen in a decade and has found enormous happiness and joy.

Post-discharge management: Josh is followed on an outpatient basis by Dr. Marotta for medication and by his Lodge social worker for therapy. He reconnects with old friends and is about to start graduate school when he dies in his sleep from a grand mal seizure. Unfortunately, people suffering from epilepsy, even when under careful medical care, suffer from a higher rate of sudden death, often due to seizures while sleeping. While devastated, Josh's family has lived with the understanding that the control of epilepsy through medication is not foolproof. Dr. Marotta attends Josh's funeral, where Josh is celebrated by friends and family who speak of his return to a happy and less isolated life. His parents still remain in contact with Dr. Marotta.

LESLIE

Leslie stays at The Lodge for five months.

- She is placed on **clozapine**, which appears helpful.

- She is **taken off clozapine** following a seizure which occurs at a low dose.

- She is sent for a consultation with a senior epilepsy specialist, based on the seizure she had on low-dose clozapine.

- Leslie is placed **again on clozapine, plus antiepileptic medication.**

- **Lamotrigine (Lamictal)** is added for seizure control and to decrease mood instability.

- **Divalproex (Depakote)** is added to lower seizure risk.

- **Oxytocin** is added to address social disconnectedness.

Leslie is **discharged to** a residential step-down program. She and her team there report that she continues to do well on her medications.

- Leslie takes classes.

- She gets a part-time job.

- She remains thoughtful, philosophically inclined, and continues to paint and write excessively. Her family is shocked by her improvement, stating that she has returned to a much earlier self.

Post-discharge management: Leslie's care has been taken over by the staff at the residential program.

The Extreme of Resistance: The "Hopeless" Cases

Sadly, some of the families whose loved ones end up as residents of The Lodge program have previously been told that there is no future for their loved one at all. They have been advised to place them in long-term institutions, to give up hope of any rescue. At The Lodge, the team avoids these "prepackaged" diagnoses and prognostic dictums; each case is a puzzle to be solved, none more or less than any other. Here, in his own words, is Dr. Marotta's perspective:

> Several members of my family served with the Seabees during World War II. These naval construction battalions had a great motto: "The difficult we do now, the impossible takes a little longer." Sometimes at The Lodge we are presented with cases on the extreme of "resistance." Sometimes we are told by the families that we are their last hope, since they have been told their situation is "hopeless" and their child will need to be institutionalized. This is an enormous challenge, not simply intellectually, testing our knowledge and reasoning powers, but also emotionally. How do we turn around hopelessness in others? How do we not become hopeless ourselves? It is a question of morale and support. It is a function of the interplay of families and team members, the institution, and of course, the patients themselves. It starts by admitting this will take time, but also clearly committing to not giving up.

Eleanor, Sidney, and Stuart are good examples of "hopeless" cases, considered lost at sea, whose time at The Lodge program proved that they were not lost after all.

ELEANOR

Eleanor stays at The Lodge for four months.

- Eleanor arrives at The Lodge because of behavior induced by brain trauma suffered from an accident. She is described by Dr. Marotta as ataxic, dysarthric, mood labile and perseverative.* Her judgment is clearly impaired, and although her IQ is still very high, she has a formal thought disorder. Eleanor, on the other hand, thinks she is doing well. "I just need Adderall and I will be fine," she says.

- **Amphetamine/dextroamphetamine (Adderall)** is added to increase her focus and concentration.

- **Risperidone (Risperdal)** is added to address her extreme emotional lability, but Eleanor is still out of control and needs to be returned to the ACU, where she is stabilized and then returned to The Lodge.

- **Lithium** is added to decrease mood instability.

- The **amphetamine/dextroamphetamine (Adderall)** dose is increased.

- Dr. Marotta's notes reflect a recognition that in addition to behavioral control of her frontal lobe syndrome, Eleanor's sense of loss surrounding her identity and life goals will need to be addressed as well. As a consequence of her accident, he writes, "Eleanor is dealing with a massive loss of self and all that she might have been. It is obvious that it will be a very difficult case to manage. It will call for a very integrated treat-

---

* Ataxia is impaired coordination; dysarthria is a disorder of speech, in this case due to brain damage; mood lability refers to frequent, unpredictable changes of emotion; perseverative thinking refers to a repetitive thought pattern that is uncontrollable.

ment plan." In fact, Eleanor gets easily frustrated and upset. She gets perseverative and gets into power struggles with the staff. Her inability to change her mindset and her early resistance to accepting her treatment plan results in another stay in the ACU. She is then returned to The Lodge.

- **Lorazepam (Ativan)** is tried but does not help.

- **Carbamazepine (Tegretol)** is added for seizure control related to her brain damage.

- The **amphetamine/dextroamphetamine (Adderall)** dose is increased again and does help.

- **Donepezil (Aricept)** is added to help with memory.

- **Fluoxetine (Prozac)** is added to address Eleanor's depression.

- **Propranolol (Inderal)** is added to address her anger and impulsiveness (discontinued by discharge).

- **Risperidone (Risperdal)** is added for mood stability (discontinued by discharge).

- **Buspirone (Buspar)** is added for anger and irritability (discontinued by discharge).

- **Liothyronine (Cytomel)** is added for hypothyroidism.

- **Vitamins** are added for nutrition.

During her stay at The Lodge, the team works hard to develop a trusting relationship with Eleanor, and her developing attachment to the treatment team proves critical to her success in the program. Her initial stay at The Lodge is characterized by power struggles and perseverative resistant behavior. The treatment team repeatedly communicates that they will not give up until they help her achieve a better life. They also actively listen to her communication and do not discount her experience because she is impaired. As she begins to trust them, the power struggles begin to decrease. Her behavior will always be somewhat perseverative because of her frontal lobe injury, so her therapists work to help her recognize her own cognitive vulnerabilities and develop coping strategies. They model behavior and she begins to copy them. For example, she mentors another resident the way she has been mentored, helping her work in the hospital store. Staff also help her to rethink her life goals and to believe a satisfying life will be possible. They maintain contact with outside consultants and institutions that will aid in TBI (traumatic brain injury) rehabilitation post-discharge in order to maintain continuity of care.

Eleanor is **discharged to** an urban apartment.

- She plans to do volunteer work.

- She works with a physical trainer.

- She takes foreign language lessons.

- She goes back to graduate school, ultimately shifting focus to studies that better accommodate her cognitive strengths.

- She falls in love and gets married.

Post-discharge management: Eleanor continues to work with Dr. Marotta and her primary social worker from The Lodge. Her connection runs deep. She paints pictures for members of Dr. Marotta's family and remembers people on their birthdays. (Read more about Eleanor's story in her own and her mother's words following this chapter).

STUART

Stuart stays at The Lodge for eight months.

- Stuart is a tortured soul. When he arrives at SHH for his first stay, he has been grossly psychotic for years and his illness has been unresponsive to treatment. He hears constant critical voices, and his acute paranoia makes him difficult to manage.

- He is placed on **clozapine** in the ACU to address acute hallucinations and delusions. Stuart's symptoms respond well to the clozapine but almost immediately his **liver enzymes become extremely elevated** ("the highest numbers I have ever seen," says Dr. Marotta), a sign that he may be at risk for clozapine-induced hepatic failure.

- The team feels they have no choice but to **stop the clozapine,** and his doctors begin a series of trials of other medicines.

- Stuart has minimal success with symptom reduction on a combination of **loxapine (Loxitane)** and **gabapentin (Neurontin)**. After close to a year in the program, his parents decide that he should be discharged to a residential setting. Outside the hospital, his paranoia gets worse.

- He is **readmitted** to SHH.

- The team at SHH **stabilizes him with haloperidol (Haldol)** and he is **discharged** again.

Stuart struggles for the next year, unable to function because of his constant voices, and ultimately returns to his parents' home, where he lives an isolated existence. Desperate, Stuart's parents approach SHH once more, and the team agrees to work with him again. Stuart's symptoms are so extreme that over the next several months he is transferred between The Lodge and the ACU multiple times.

- Based on his past history, the team does not initially place Stuart on clozapine but begins a **series of trials of different medications** and medication combinations. Unfortunately, his critical voices and paranoia remain, making him exceedingly unstable and at times a danger to himself or others.

- The team discusses his case repeatedly and **finally decides that starting him on clozapine again is his only chance for a reasonable life.** They discuss the risks with Stuart and Stuart's parents, and all agree that the team should proceed despite the risks. The smallest clozapine tablet is 25 mg. **The team decides to divide a 25 mg tablet into four pieces, and to move Stuart's dose up in 6+ mg increments.** Blood work is monitored closely following each incremental change. The team reviews the case constantly, as they are taking an enormous risk.

- The team thinks they see an inflection point in Stuart's improvement when they get him to a blood level of clozapine over 300. Over nearly a year's time, the team continues to raise the dose slowly, and they note a continuing reduction in his hallucinations and paranoia. His liver enzymes remain in a tolerable zone.

- He is placed on **lurasidone (Latuda) and haloperidol (Haldol)** to address residual psychotic symptoms, while his clozapine dose is being slowly raised.

- After further discussion, he is placed on **duloxetine (Cymbalta)** to address depression and obsessiveness.

- He is placed on **lorazepam (Ativan)** to address anxiety.

- The team places him on **oxytocin** to address continuing issues with social connection. This addition helps him interact with other people. Stuart reports that together, clozapine and oxytocin give him enormous relief. Dr. Marotta notes, "He began strolling the halls, coming to his doctors' offices to tell them how things were going and giving them the occasional hug." In fact, Stuart's relationship with all the staff at The Lodge becomes very close. "He became like a family member," says Dr. Marotta.

Stuart describes his medication experience:

The clozapine relieved my paranoia. I'm not constantly looking over my shoulder. My mind is moving at a smoother pace, not too fast or too slow. It does knock me out. But the result is totally worth it. Latuda helped me have a brighter outlook on life. It gave me a significant mood boost the first couple of weeks—less now—probably because of the Haldol. I'm more mellow and calmer. I thought Cymbalta was the magical drug about a year ago, but I'm not sure I feel anything now. I guess it is to be debated. Ativan perhaps helps me feel more calm—at ease—helps me settle into groups. And with Oxytocin, it feels easier to talk to people.

Overall, he says, "I really feel good. I am looking forward to being with the family. The medications are really working well, and I feel we have a really good mix. The voices are nearly gone, and I can control them. I feel happy and good. I appreciate all you have done."

Stuart is **discharged to** a rural residential community, where he has a happy multi-month stay before returning to his parents' home.

- Stuart moves to his own apartment in an urban environment. While his voices have not totally disappeared, he says medication allows him to ignore them.

- He joins a men's support group.

- He works at part-time jobs and is able to enjoy his life.

Post-discharge management: Stuart continues a supportive relationship with his doctors from The Lodge program, seeing his psychiatrist weekly in their outpatient practice. It is a life still limited, but now not overwhelmed by psychotic illness. It is a far cry from life in an institution, and one that would not have occurred without the patience and persistence of Stuart, his parents, and all the staff involved. Dr. Marotta says, "The decrease in PANSS from 130 to 44 is a shadow of the enormous change in Stuart's life. He is actively engaged in life and hopeful for his future. Finding the right medications, albeit a complex mix, compliance, and sobriety are central to this miracle." It is truly a life reimagined.

SIDNEY

Sidney stays at the ACU for two months, where he is managed by The Lodge team; he then stays at The Lodge for six months.

- Sidney is brought to SHH's ACU from across the country by an interventionist. He has a long history of multiple hospitalizations, with only one period of sustained residential treatment amidst a sea of psychotic decompensations. Because of his extreme level of impairment and noncompliance, at various points his parents were advised to place him on the wait list for a long-term locked unit or let him live in a homeless shelter and leave his care to the state. A Covid infection has entirely destabilized him again, and he arrives poorly groomed, internally preoccupied, perseverative, and paranoid. Physical exam also reveals a significant wound, which is clearly infected. He is immediately sent to a local hospital for medical attention.

- When he returns to SHH, Sidney is **stabilized on the ACU. He is back on clozapine** (which he had taken previously), but his early behavior at The Lodge is disorganized and poorly related. He isolates himself, has poor self-care, mumbles or laughs to himself, shadowboxes unseen opponents, and seems to argue with others who are not there. His doctor sees him as sweet, but his behavior appears intimidating to others who don't know him. He has practically no capacity to relate to other residents in the milieu and has extremely limited ability to relate to the team.

- The **staff takes their cues from Sidney**, giving him space and observing. Sidney's family is extremely supportive of both Sidney and the team, allowing the team time to begin the process of an extensive assessment of both psychiatric and physical symptoms.

- Consultants are contacted to assess Sidney's physical wound, which has failed to heal completely, and the team **considers the possibility of an autoimmune component** to this continuing problem.

- He is placed on **low-dose levothyroxine (Synthroid)** to address mild hypothyroidism.

- **Haloperidol (Haldol)** is added to address his acute positive symptoms of schizophrenia.

- **Divalproex (Depakote)** is added to decrease seizure risk.

- **Donepezil (Aricept)** is added to stimulate cognition and decrease concrete thinking.*

- **Propranolol (Inderal)** is added to address a high pulse rate, which may stem from either his chronic wound infection or a medication he is taking.

- **Oxytocin** is added to address Sidney's emotional disconnection.

- **Clonazepam (Klonopin)** is added to address his anxiety.

- He is placed on **medications to address a variety of physical issues, including wound care and excess salivation.**

---

* Concrete thinking means an inability to understand abstract concepts or connection. If you exhibit concrete thinking you cannot easily change your mindset, making it difficult to accept an alternative view of reality.

- He is placed on **vitamins, such as methylfolate (Deplin), and supplements** to help with nutrition.

- With gentle support, Sidney continues to take his medication and begins to show slow but steady signs of improvement over the course of months. Developing a connection to others takes time. He has been acutely ill for years, and it takes time for his paranoia and internal preoccupations to decrease. The staff is patient. Initially, all Sidney can tolerate is standing side by side with a residential counselor. Slowly, things change. He can look his favorite staff member in the eye for one second, and then two. Sidney develops a particular attachment to a few team members, who work to gently extend Sidney's ability to interact and communicate his thoughts. They learn his likes and dislikes, and their ability to anticipate and adapt to his needs forms the basis of his developing trust and willingness to follow their guidance.

- Sidney's **clozapine dose is raised over time to a high level**, keeping his blood levels in the extremely high thera-peutic range. But he has tolerated it well. The team discusses the decision to continue him at this high level with Sidney's family, and all agree that the benefits outweigh the risks. His acute symptoms are noticeably better. He is less agitated, better able to take care of himself with reminders and has slowly become able to communicate with other residents and participate in the milieu. He is now accepted by his peers. He begins to have numerous outings with his family, which he thoroughly enjoys.

- **After six months, discharge plans are initiated**. He has become less paranoid and more related and less bothered by internal voices. While some chronic behaviors remain, these are less intense and less frequent. Although his thinking is still somewhat concrete, he now expresses his thoughts and desires, and his sense of agency has increased. For example, when shopping with his mother for clothes, he is concerned with making a good impression on others. Sidney now under-stands that his behavior and presentation make an impact on the world around him. He is anxious about leaving The Lodge, but he is willing to try. Sidney's wound is still an issue, but it has been controlled while he has been at SHH. Now that he is more stable, the team will help his family investigate further treatment.

Sidney is **discharged** to a rural residential community. His dream has been to work and receive a paycheck. While contemplating discharge, Sidney's family collaborates with the team and listens to recommendations from other Lodge alum parents. They take him on a couple of visits to the small residential program which they feel can best accommodate his needs and desires. Sidney's visits go well, and he is happy that he will know a couple of people at the program. Sidney is discharged and his family reports that he is thriving. A new surgical team is engaged, and after procedures and antibiotics his wound heals.

- Sidney works part-time.

- He lives in a supervised apartment.

- He is happy and socially engaging when his former Lodge team comes to visit.

Post-discharge management: Sidney's parents remain in contact with Dr. Marotta, but his day-to-day psychiatric needs are overseen by local mental health-care providers who have a collaborative relationship with The Lodge program. He is stable enough to finally undergo additional medical procedures which are necessary for long-term health. Post-surgeries, his psychiatric status has improved remarkably, leading Dr. Marotta to suspect that his chronic infection has had a larger impact on his psychiatric illness than would have been suspected from a conventional perspective. He is living a life that he imagined. For his family, thoughts of his future are no longer filled with despair. (Sidney's mother's moving account of their story can be found following Chapter Four.)

PUTTING IT ALL TOGETHER

Finding an optimally successful medication regimen for someone struggling with NBD is an ongoing process and must begin with a full and detailed evaluation. The benefit of a longer stay in a hospital program is that a truer understanding of the contributing factors of a patient's NBD can be developed, and initial medication trials and changes can take place in a safely supervised environment. The importance of time for the process of evaluation and medication adjustment, regardless of where it takes place, cannot be overstated. As can be seen from the examples in this chapter, individuals have different responses to the same medications, and similar symptoms can have different root causes. Medication prescriptions based solely on initial diagnosis can be limited in their efficacy, and particularly in cases of persistent psychosis there are many factors that need to be considered.

This chapter points to the patience and time necessary when trying to find the right balance of medications, and to the importance of having a sustaining relationship with clinicians who can keep you going during this process. It also highlights the importance of persistence and hope in finding interventions that address both the positive and negative symptoms of NBD. Particularly after discharge, unpredictable life events can threaten vulnerabilities or, alternatively, foster greater stability. Additionally, the cumulative effects of medication over time and the illness itself impact vulnerable systems and require periodic recalibration of medication regimes and reevaluation of overall treatment plans. A good captain and crew do not hesitate to rechart the ship's course if a wind blows it sideways. Course correction is a fundamental part of arriving at your destination.

KEY IDEAS FOR CHAPTER SIX:
CHARTING THE COURSE

- **Attention needs to be paid to possible effects of medical conditions** (e.g., seizure disorders, autoimmune disorders, infections); consultants should be called in when necessary.

- **Medication adjustment is a necessary part of the recovery process.** In these complex cases, with possible multiple underlying pathophysiological processes at work, polypharmacy is often necessary for long-term success and requires the close management of highly trained teams of specialists (similar to the treatment of cancer or diabetes by highly trained oncology and nephrology specialists).

- **Symptoms should be addressed individually;** remember, side effects can result from medication as well as illness.

- **Staff need to listen carefully to patients' experiences;** e.g., patient use of certain substances may be a clue to underlying processes, not just addictive behavior.

- **No case is viewed as hopeless.** It is important to accept that difficult cases may take more time but outcome goals remain the same.

- **Case management post-discharge is individualized and essential to continued recovery.** Even when management is transferred to other providers, it should be communicated that the door to the program staff and treatment remains open to both patients and their families if down the line they wish to reconnect and return.

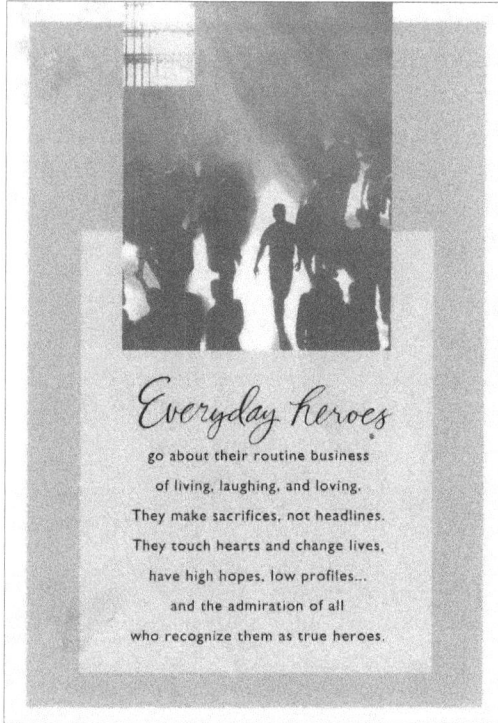

FIGURE 4: *Outside of Eleanor's Card to Dr. Marotta*

Source: Card sent to Dr. Marotta by Eleanor.

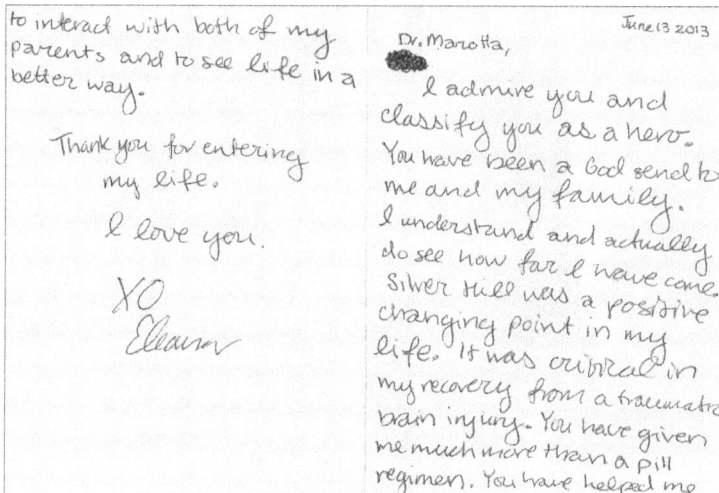

to interact with both of my
parents and to see life in a
better way.

Thank you for entering
my life.

I love you.

XO
Eleanor

June 13 2013

Dr. Marotta,

I admire you and
classify you as a hero.
You have been a God send to
me and my family.
I understand and actually
do see how far I have come.
Silver Hill was a positive
changing point in my
life. It was critical in
my recovery from a traumatic
brain injury. You have given
me much more than a pill
regimen. You have helped me

FIGURE 5: *Inside of Eleanor's Card to Dr. Marotta*

Source: Card sent to Dr. Marotta by Eleanor.

ELEANOR
—An Alum's Story*

Five years, three months, and twenty-nine days ago, I fell more than twenty feet headfirst into rocks and incurred a severe traumatic brain injury. To add insult to injury, I had been intending to jump into the water. So, after my body hit the ground, I slid into the water, and I started to drown.

For the first year of my recovery, I could not feel emotions as one normally is able to do, so writing down my thoughts helped me to express my emotions. To get to the heart of the matter, the biggest difference in life for me after my brain injury was my lack of emotions. As my emotions began to return, I found I was not able to control them. I was not in a good place.

Very fortunately, one of my problem behaviors led to a blessing. In September of 2011, I was caught by the pharmacy for forging the prescription of a controlled substance. The only way charges would not be pressed against me was if I enrolled in a program for mental illness or addiction.

After we found Silver Hill Hospital, I went there to be interviewed and my mother stepped in to give an explanation of my case. Truth be told, my mother literally cried to Dr. Marotta and begged him to admit me. Against their better judgment, the hospital agreed to take me. I was in a bad place when I arrived in New Canaan. I had lost all the independence I had slowly regained since my traumatic brain injury, I could not control my emotions, and frankly, I did not want to be alive. More than anything, what I gained from my stay at Silver Hill was an appreciation of life.

From my time at Silver Hill to this day, I consider myself having two sets of parents. One being my biological and step-family. The other being my medical family: my mother is social worker Lisa Goldenberg and my father is neuropsychiatrist Dr. Rocco Marotta. They showered me with attention and concern while they worked to help me recover during my time at the hospital.

Silver Hill Hospital made me a more complete person. I became sober, shaped up physically, centered my emotions, had the correct medication formulated for me, and regained my confidence in myself. To conclude, I must reiterate that during my stay, I relearned to love being alive.

Rocco Marotta, MD, PhD. He would not give up and would not let me give up.

---

* Adapted from a 2016 speech at the Silver Hill Hospital Gala.

MY DAUGHTER, ELEANOR
—A Parent's Story

My daughter was beautiful. She was smart, with a quick wit. Funny and kind, long legs and big brown eyes. When she graduated from Undergraduate Business School at UNC Chapel Hill in 2008, she decided she was really meant to be a doctor. So she enrolled in the post-baccalaureate premed school at Columbia University to take courses to apply to medical school.

During the summer after completing the first year, her world collapsed. She slipped and fell thirty feet from a tree onto the rocky shore of the pond into which she intended to jump. (She was also athletic and fearless.)

Three weeks later she awoke from a coma. Her head was shaved, with a scar spanning across the top from ear to ear from a craniotomy (a front skull flap was temporarily removed due to brain swelling and stored in the abdomen, which also had a long scar). The recovery from this frontal lobe brain injury began.

A year later we sat in the admitting lobby of Silver Hill Hospital. Eleanor was agitated and furious about being there. After her interview, it was my turn to see the doctor in charge. I sat across from Dr. Rocco Marotta as he explained that SHH did not treat traumatic brain injury patients. He had studied them at Yale and was knowledgeable in the area of frontal lobe function.

I lost all composure and fell into a state of hysteria. We had researched and visited TBI residential centers across the US. Nowhere could we find a fit for her needs. Every TBI is different, as the brain is a complex miracle of specialized zones and interconnections that modern science only minimally understands. It is known the frontal lobes govern personality, executive function, impulse control, recent memory. She suffered symptoms of each. How much recovery would be possible, and how could she be helped?

It's unclear whether Dr Marotta decided to bend the admission policy because of his past training or to console the sobbing mother sitting in front of him. Whatever the reason, it was a lifesaving decision for one beautiful young woman and her family.

I was living nearby in Pound Ridge, a quick drive to Silver Hill in New Canaan. I could visit frequently to provide support and was for-

Continued ➤

tunate to share the experience of her slow progress. Initially, she was unable to control emotions and outbursts, and lost privileges. The counselors were patient. There were group therapies, and she could visit the exercise building. She began forming relationships with other residents of The Lodge.

From the beginning, Eleanor developed a strong respect for the busy doctor who was treating her. Dr Marotta made her laugh and talked about his own daughter. He carefully prescribed a succession of meds, discussing each, encouraging her feedback, and monitoring her treatment. I observed that, though her challenges resulted from a TBI, other residents shared similar personality differences. Perhaps they are governed by the same areas of the brain and respond to similar pharmacological treatment. She received quite knowledgeable care.

Lisa Goldenberg, a Senior Social Worker and her Primary Therapist, became a lifeline and confidant, whose office was always open. I was able to meet with both Dr. M. and Lisa and other staff. Never was I treated with indifference or as an intruder. I felt we were all working to help my daughter.

Our family was fortunate to be able to afford the cost of extending the SHH residency beyond the customary thirty days. It was crucial to have time for observation and adjustment to [determine] the effective mix of drugs. The various therapies, support groups, and behavior modifications entail a slow building process. Any brain treatment needs time, time, time.

For five months she resided and recovered at Silver Hill. Importantly, she was able to continue as a private patient with Dr. Marotta as she next attended the Brain Injury Day Program at the Rusk Institute at NYU, which lasted twenty weeks.

The following fall she returned to Columbia University. During that time she was invited to be the featured speaker at the Silver Hill Gala, receiving a standing ovation from the 600 guests.

Columbia's premed program now proved to be too rigorous, but she met another student and fell in love. They married later in August of 2016. Lisa and Rocco Marotta and Lisa and Dave Goldenberg traveled to North Carolina to attend the wedding.

She remained a patient of Dr. Marotta and called him her "second Father."

That December, she was driving home from a medical appointment, collapsed at the wheel, and was in a fatal single-car accident.

Eleanor's story is both a triumph and a tragedy, and, like Josh's tragic death, underscores the variety of ways in which despite our best attempts, control over all of life's variables is impossible. Eleanor's accident was caused by an unexpected physical response to a medical procedure (she fainted while driving), totally unrelated to her Lodge treatment. She was happy and reengaged in her life, optimistic and excited about her future.

Eleanor's memory is cherished by all who knew her. To this day, her family remains connected to some of the team members.

Chapter 7

DENIAL OF ILLNESS

"Every man takes the limits of his own field of vision for the limits of the world."

—*Arthur Schopenhauer*

"There are many truths of which the full meaning cannot be realized until personal experience has brought it home."

—*John Stuart Mill*

THE PROBLEM OF DENIAL

It is inspiring and important to write about the remarkable transformations that can occur for individuals with severe neuropsychiatric disorders as the result of persistent, caring, and integrated treatment.[1] Stories of returning to school and graduating with advanced degrees, attaining successful professional lives, and developing the ability to find love and marriage are welcome antidotes to our historically dark predictions of lives totally unraveled, cognitive decline, and hopeless outcomes. It is equally compelling to feel frustration and rage when systems fail those whose recovery was interrupted because support was lacking or inadequate, where families and patients desired help but could not access appropriate treatment. But what about loved ones whose greatest obstacle to a fuller recovery is their own perspective, their inability or unwillingness to recognize that they are ill at all?

Reconnecting with one's potential requires both objective, external support, and subjective, internal intent or cooperation. Lack of insight about one's impaired functioning restricts this subjective perspective, limiting the extent to which a person can recognize the importance of various treatment interventions. This is further complicated when someone has a chronic illness with acute and dormant symptom phases. For the majority of patients with NBD, denial of illness is part of the initial symptom presentation, but with medication and supportive treatment, many will acquiesce to initial treatment, allowing acute symptoms to recede. Once acute symptoms have diminished, however, more than a few will say, "I am cured." Others will acquiesce to a longer course of treatment, but ultimately the urge to live a "normal" life free of medication and supervision will challenge their willingness to continue advised medication and treatment interventions. Denial of illness is not stoicism or the ability to compartmentalize. Individuals who are stoic soldier on, accepting the pain of their difficulty but not dwelling on its presence. Those who compartmentalize are aware of their struggle but choose to separate it from their everyday consciousness, accessing its existence only when necessary or when it will not interfere with their functioning. Denial of illness is neither of these.

This chapter is dedicated to the dilemma of denial of illness, which, unlike stoicism or compartmentalization, exists outside of conscious control. For many patients with NBD, it will be part of the symptom picture for at least the early phase of their struggle. For others, it is a dogged part of the symptom picture for more of their journey. For any patient, there may be more than one interrelated reason for their unwillingness to accept a diagnosis of NBD, often requiring patience and a longer-term strategy to tease apart and address these factors. In fact, it is this complexity of reasons for denial of illness that makes a multifaceted approach to treatment so critical.

Let us start with three case examples, take a closer look at the layers that can result in denial of illness in NBD, and discuss how they can be approached.

Case #1: Andrew

Andrew arrived at SHH following a near-fatal suicide attempt that required many weeks of medical hospitalization at a different facility. In an attempt to quiet tormenting voices and to avoid pursuing murderous entities, he sought to take his own life. This was not Andrew's first hospitalization for psychotic illness. In another hospitalization for a previous psychotic episode, he had been placed on clozapine, and this had allowed him to return to work and graduate school following discharge. But post-hospitalization, he had taken himself off medication because he felt he no longer needed it.

In this current hospitalization, back on a complex mixture of medications, including clozapine, he was better again but consistently ambivalent about taking medication in general. While acknowledging that his paranoia, ambivalence, social withdrawal, and concrete thinking were slowly decreasing, Andrew was still not sure whether his classic signs of schizophrenia were due to illness or had been the result of the negative effects of previous medication.

Following his hospitalization at SSH, Andrew returned to work again, but he felt his work performance had decreased and blamed this on medication side effects. Despite persuasive evidence, Andrew does not see himself as schizophrenic and is frustrated that taking medicine makes him tired, limits drinking, and prevents him from engaging in the kind of social experience he feels is necessary and desirable for work and social life in general. He avoids many of his scheduled meetings with his psychiatrist and therapist and seems to have forgotten about the intensity of his previous psychotic symptoms that have resulted in his three hospitalizations. Despite worsening symptoms as he takes less and less medication, Andrew does not accept that he has an NBD illness. His parents and his psychiatrist continue to collaborate, while Andrew continues to resist. His denial of illness may now be the biggest obstacle to his own continued recovery.

CASE #2: LEO*

Leo, now middle-aged, has been inconsistent with his medication for years. While he once held a job, following repeated hospitalizations, he no longer works and has lost most of his friends. When hospitalized he is medication-compliant, but when he is discharged his belief that he is

---

* Leo is a composite case, made up of a number of case elements from patients with whom Dr. Marotta has worked.

not really ill erodes his willingness to take his prescribed clozapine. His family has been unable to persuade him that his life will be better if he takes this medication. They have barely been able to get him to accept injectable antipsychotics, which they have made a requirement of their financial support.

Leo, who seemed destined for great achievement throughout his childhood, now lives a relatively marginal life. He has no job, occasionally sees family but spends most of his time alone and is disengaged from activities. He continues to smoke both cigarettes and marijuana. When asked, he rationalizes his problems. Despite clear evidence of his dysfunction, he still does not believe that he is ill.

Case #3: Sonia*

Sonia was admitted to SHH and other hospitals in the New York region on multiple occasions and was given many diagnoses. Her erratic behavior had begun early in puberty, and she had been using marijuana and alcohol since early in high school. Over time her behavior had become more provocative, with sexual adventures, substance use binges and overdoses, and a nearly fatal suicide attempt. Her family was fragmenting under the stress of her behavior and multiple failed interventions.

When she arrived at SHH, it was the team's opinion that she was actually suffering from schizoaffective disorder and was resistant to conventional interventions. The Lodge team elected to try clozapine and later added oxytocin to her medication regimen. Sonia improved remarkably over several months and was transferred to a nationally known long-term residential program. She continued to do so well that her new team at the residential program did not accept The Lodge team's view of her case. They felt she was not psychotically ill, and Sonia embraced this perspective. Against The Lodge team advice, the new team stopped her medications and changed the focus of treatment to personality disorder and substance abuse. After a month off clozapine and oxytocin, she left the program and two weeks later died by suicide. We consider this a case of culturally supported denial of illness in favor of a less-stigmatizing diagnosis.

---

* Sonia is a composite of three cases of Lodge alumni.

THE NEUROBIOLOGY OF DENIAL OF ILLNESS: ANOSOGNOSIA

The neurological literature describes denial of illness as anosognosia. In 1914, the eminent French neurologist Joseph Babinski coined this term to describe patients suffering from an inability to recognize physical or perceptual limitations following brain trauma-induced hemiplegia (paralysis of one side of the body). Anosognosia in the context of this type of physical brain injury is more clearly correlated to specific and measurable brain lesions. For example, the imaging of a patient with a lack of awareness of perceptual or motor deficits on the left side of the body might show a clear lesion in the right parietal lobe.

With NBD, one-to-one correlations like this have yet to be found, in part because psychotic illness is not a singular disease with a simple, localized pathophysiology, and in part because research suggests complex cellular and biochemical origins. Nonetheless, the biological basis of diseases like schizophrenia is clear and for many NBD patients denial of illness is a symptom of biological (versus psychological) dysfunction.

Several recent books contain direct and important discussions of denial of illness. These include Jeffrey Lieberman, MD's *Malady of the Mind: Schizophrenia and the Path to Prevention*, E. Fuller Torrey's *Surviving Schizophrenia: A Family Manual, Seventh Edition*, and Xavier Amador, PhD's book *I Am Not Sick I Don't Need Help!: How to Help Someone Accept Treatment*, all of which have detailed some of the particulars of this complex biological issue. Imaging studies and studies of the neuroscience of "brain architecture" have all shown biological pathology in patients with schizophrenia. Reduction of brain tissue integrity and volume in different areas of the brain have been found in this population, as has disruption of dendritic connective pathways in the brain.[2]

Anosognosia that occurs in NBD is now seen, at its root, as a biologically based symptom of complex brain pathology which interferes with accurate processing of sensory, visual, and behavioral information. It is also exacerbated by the concreteness and rigidity of cognition, which is another symptom of frontal lobe brain dysfunction often seen in NBD patients and prevents patients from easily changing their perspective. Paranoia and delusions also often reinforce biologically based denial of illness. Medication compliance for those struggling with NBD addresses this biological component by impacting brain chemistry, but addressing the biology alone is not enough.

Psychological Factors in Denial of Illness

While the word "anosognosia" is often used in discussions of NBD as an overarching term to indicate general denial of illness, it is helpful to distinguish the more biologically based anosognosia from the more psychological, defensively based denial, a psychological strategy which involves the conscious or preconscious attempt to protect oneself from the negative impact of perceived or actual damaging experience. We all know the denial of illness that can prevent us from taking care of our physical problems in a timely manner, how anxiety and fear can prevent us from going to the doctor to check something out, even though we know we should. "It's probably nothing," we say to ourselves, "I feel fine." Anxiety about facing what might be wrong prevents us from making wise decisions, something we often regret with the wisdom of hindsight.

With NBD—especially in situations where an individual has shown enormous potential in early life—it can be particularly painful to face developing limitations which challenge expectations of success and the hope for a productive and satisfying future. Attempts to ward off the emotional impact of this hurt can come in the form of partial or full denial of illness by both patients and their families. And after having weathered a crisis, subsequent periods of increased stability are also vulnerable times for many individuals with NBD. Feeling better, the pull to be "normal" is strong, leading patients to reduce or stop their medication and/or resume their use of substances, despite advice that this may negate the progress they've made. This type of denial can be seen as part of a struggle to affirm the primacy of self and freedom. This is understandable in a culture so committed to individual expression and autonomy. Psychological defenses can be layered on top of the propensity for biologically based anosognosia, and for some patients, it is the major impediment to owning their diagnosis.

Let us tease this apart further. Not all defensive, psychological denial of illness is triggered by the same causes. Human behavior is complicated. The expression of genetic, biochemical, and neurological vulnerabilities are filtered through individual temperament and personality variables and impacted additionally by environment and individual history. Psychological factors in denial of illness similarly reflect these differences in variables. Why is this important? Because strategies for intervention may be overtly or subtly directed by an understanding of which of these factors are particularly central to someone's defensive denial. For example, denial of illness may stem from:

- worry about survival: "How could anyone continue to live and function with these problems?"*

- confusion about what is happening: "I used to be able to do X,Y, Z. How could I not be able to do them now?"

- narcissistic grandiosity: "I have an important life and work, so I can't possibly be limited by dysfunction."

- desire to feel special or chosen: "I am a chosen one and my differences are not problems but reflect my special status."

- worry about being different: "Who am I if I am not like family and friends, and don't fit into the norm of society? I just want to be like everyone else, just a regular person."

- paranoid belief that an external threat as opposed to an internal illness is at the root of my difficulties: "I am struggling because people are against me and throwing obstacles in my way."

While more than one of these factors may be in play, identifying the predominant psychological experience of someone's resistance can be critical, especially when deciding on initial approaches to treatment.

SOCIOCULTURAL ISSUES IN DENIAL OF ILLNESS

To make matters still more complicated, there are sociocultural factors that must be taken into consideration and can reinforce an individual's denial of illness. Although not all cultures perceive mental illness in the same

---

* The Lodge team has speculated that there may even be an evolutionary pull for defensive denial, i.e., that denial of impairment may be supported by the human species' need to soldier on if they are to survive.

way, the negative stigma attached to mental illness in our Western culture should not be overlooked. As stated clearly by Elyn Saks, an associate dean and Professor of Law, Psychology, and Psychiatry and the Behavioral Sciences at the University of Southern California Gould Law School, who herself carries a diagnosis of schizophrenia, "Mental illness carries a huge stigma. Even people who do not purposely deny the illness they know they have may unconsciously do so for the very same reason as the conscious deniers. One brings shame upon oneself, so to speak, by admitting to the illness."[3] In the majority of cases, the stereotype of mental illness portrayed in popular movies or in the media is one of disorganized dysfunction at best, and violent instability of thought and behavior at worst. Who would want to be associated with that? Alternative explanations for why your problems are occurring would be highly preferable.

Ironically, the other stereotype of mental illness in Western culture revolves around the opposite perspective—a romanticized view of the tortured mind. This can also reinforce the denial of illness. Dramatic stories of poets and artists associate struggles with deep depression and mania with genius, and writings about holy persons with eccentricities, isolated behavior, and visions sanctify these attributes. Delusional systems of individuals with NBD sometimes involve the belief that they have been chosen in some fashion. Perhaps they are chosen by a deity or are the deity themselves. Perhaps they have special talents. The fact that throughout our history we have celebrated the madness of certain individuals can reinforce the idea that what others call symptoms are in fact not illness but a sign of specialness. Who wouldn't want that?

Approaches to Working with Denial of Illness

How, then, should denial of illness be approached by both families and providers? Dr. Marotta and The Lodge team believe that the complicated nature of denial of illness in NBD makes it necessary to take a multifaceted approach to intervention. Medication is necessary to address biologically based anosognosia because the ability to process and make sense of information accurately requires intervention at biochemical and cellular levels. Cognitive interventions help to shift thinking. Psychodynamically oriented* conversation helps individuals understand their symptoms as part of a life narrative which has had adaptive meaning.[4] It is important to understand, however, that changing a person's mindset requires patience. Rarely do these kinds of changes happen immediately, and it is part of a clinician's role to help families understand when to challenge and when to hold back.

How can you develop a connection to someone who doesn't want to hear or believe what you want to convey? Here is Dr. Marotta's and The Lodge team's advice:

- **Establishing a rapport is essential.** It means listening to and respecting your loved one's perception of reality. The more someone feels respected, the more likely they are to share their true experience. As this experience is revealed, it is important to try and identify issues that they themselves may find troubling. Especially when delusions and hallucinations are most virulent, a patient may recognize that they are having difficulty with related issues like focus or concentration, even if they deny that it is due to illness. Once a trusting relationship with providers is developed, "cognitive errors can be gently corrected," says Dr. Marotta. "I always listen carefully to my patients and acknowledge the possibility of their experience before I try to plant doubt or alternative explanations. I might say, 'It could be, but it also could not be,' or 'I've had strange experiences too, so I know they are possible, but it is easier to believe, for example, that the deity is working through you than that you are the deity.'"

- **Making sure you understand the true nature of your loved one's psychotic symptoms is vital**. Therefore, getting a good diagnostic evaluation is key. Use whatever hook you can to initiate participation. What constitutes a good diagnostic evaluation? Dr. Marotta says, "Don't rely on evaluations that are based on statistical 'color coding' or ideology. A good evaluation looks carefully at nuance and gray areas. It looks for individual idiosyncrasies rather than statistical averages." In Chapter Six for instance, the Zebra case studies highlight

---

* Psychodynamics focuses on the conscious and unconscious thoughts and emotions that influence behavior.

how patients' seemingly "problematic" behavior (i.e., taking benzodiazepines) was reinterpreted as more "understandable" behavior (i.e., it decreased seizure-related symptoms) based on the results of a more extensive evaluation. Careful evaluation is particularly important in an age when young people are exposed to a variety of drugs and experiences with risk of toxic consequences for brain development and behavior.

- **If, after evaluation, it is clear that your loved one is suffering from psychotic illness, then the first step is to engage them in a collaborative experience of treatment.** "We always admit that we, the medical-psychiatric team, have a particular worldview," says Dr. Marotta. "We 'cop' to the charge that we see things in terms of a particular Western, medical/scientific perspective, and that in this paradigm one might see us as 'agents of state oppression.' We admit to that and then appeal to our patients' empathy towards us, and hope that they can come to appreciate our struggle to 'do good and be helpful.' To do this we must be present and real, appreciated as competent, and not work simply from within the role of authority. To paraphrase an old Alcoholics Anonymous saying, we want to communicate that we are all 'bozos on this bus,' and we all need to learn along the way." Getting an individual to engage in collaborative treatment does not necessarily depend on their acceptance of a specific diagnosis. The earlier and longer someone is medication-compliant and engaged in treatment, the more time their brain has to heal and for perspective to develop. Working with a provider who is invested in a long-term relationship and can help you navigate the ebb and flow of treatment compliance is particularly important.

- **Wherever possible, engage your loved one with facts.** Many of us find challenges to our way of thinking more persuasive if there is data to support the argument we are hearing. Conveying to your loved one that it is not just your opinion but that there is actual scientific evidence to support taking medication and abstaining from substance use may be helpful. For example, it is important to communicate that research has shown that psychosis is the expression of portions of the central nervous system failing and repeated episodes can lead to changes that may be irreversible and progress over time.[5] Data also support the fact that fewer and shorter episodes of psychosis predict improved long-term outcomes of the illness.[6] Therefore, behavior and medication that can mitigate or reverse states of psychosis are clearly beneficial. Some medications, such as clozapine or clozapine in conjunction with lithium, may even be protective against further damage to the central nervous system. Conversely, taking neurotoxic agents that lead to triggering or worsening states of psychosis, such as cannabis and methamphetamines, should be avoided. The data that links increasing use of cannabis and stimulants to increasing rates of psychosis in teenagers and young adults is an important piece of information about which your loved one should know.[7] Some important international studies about this subject are referenced in the Appendix.

- **Do not underestimate the issue of medication side effects as an aspect of more general resistance to diagnosis and treatment**. If your loved one is initially ambivalent about taking medication, problems with side effects can reinforce this resistance. For example, clozapine, the most effective antipsychotic, has side effects that are difficult to tolerate for some patients and may be resisted. How is this handled at The Lodge? First, Dr. Marotta and the team acknowledge the seriousness of their patients' feedback. Especially in the early stages of treatment, patients tend to be more focused on their present experience than long-term goals. It is the job of staff to present and reinforce the longer-term perspective. It is also important to remind patients that the intensity of side effects may be temporary. Second, titrating medication upward very slowly and in small increments sometimes helps soften side effects. Third, medications and strategies to counter side effects are also used and continually assessed and reassessed for effectiveness. Dr. Marotta notes:

In my opinion, reliance on "evidence-based," short, placebo-controlled medication trials is often misplaced when one is faced with real-world, severely ill neuropsychiatric cases, because [those trials] are focused on a statistical average versus individual response to medications. Multiple medications and complex interventions are often necessary, as well as the willingness to listen, to rethink, and to replan, sometimes repeatedly. When I consider using a medication to control symptoms, I am only concerned about what might be most effective in each particular case. Decisions to try a different medication to address symptoms that have not resolved are based on my assessment of the possible biological mechanisms underlying a problem as well as the full history of a patient. It is usually clear, listening to the patient, the staff, and family, whether or not something is effective once tried.

Chapter Six's case study of Stuart provides an illustration of the interplay between all these elements.

- **Understanding the full and detailed history of an individual's life is an essential tool in deciding how to approach denial of illness.** Understanding if someone is consciously rationalizing behavior requires a long view of their previous experiences. If Dr. Marotta has a long-standing relationship with a patient and believes they are consciously manipulating information, he may choose to challenge them directly (e.g., "Either you are full of bulls*t or you are very ill," he tells one patient he has worked with for almost a decade who is rationalizing his use of substances despite spiraling downward). Understanding the full history also allows him to serve as a working memory for a patient who, caught up in the present moment, doesn't remember the consequences of past behavior and experience (e.g., "Remember how bad things got the last time you started smoking weed," he tells another. "You ended up in the hospital.").

- **Immersion in a peer community where others are actively engaged in their own treatment is often extremely helpful in softening someone's denial of illness**. Watching other people who have accepted their diagnosis and are progressing toward a meaningful life is often more persuasive than someone telling you what to do. You may be resisting a diagnosis, but if you see someone similar to you getting more and more control over their own life, this sends a powerful message. The key is to find a community where individuals are actively working toward rebuilding their lives. Continue to advocate for your loved one's participation in groups where community members are at different stages of treatment. "Our patients are often the best advocates for each other," says Dr. Marotta. "They are also great examples for what is sometimes possible. We are not like a boot camp trying to weed out recruits, but like a school trying to find a way to bring all to their maximum level of possible achievement."

Fountain House—which operates under the clubhouse model* of support for those struggling with brain illness and associated difficulties, such as lack of housing and employment—features a different approach to working with psychotic illness but shares The Lodge's belief in the power of peer connection and community relationship. "Members" of Fountain House work alongside staff to accomplish the tasks involved in the daily operation of the clubhouse. They are not pushed to accept diagnoses or accept medication, although it is offered along with crisis intervention, but they are often a strong source of feedback to each other. This can be a motivator for change.

- **If your loved one continues to reject "best advice," take a break but never give up!** Stuart's case is a good example of persistence. Denial of illness and resistance to treatment, as we have discussed, can be multifaceted and complicated. Sometimes it is necessary to remove yourself from the power struggle. But over time, an individual's viewpoint may modulate or be affected by lived history, resulting in compromise and slowly decreasing resistance. For example, getting your loved one to take even small amounts of medication may alter their brain chemistry enough to allow them to question the reality of their delusions. Or actions taken off medication may lead to such frightening consequences that a

---

* A clubhouse is a community-based location designed to support the recovery of people living with serious mental illness. The concept of a clubhouse is that community is therapy.

person may reconsider taking medication. Conversations may uncover reasons for resistance which, when understood more clearly, can be addressed by providers with cognitive and psychodynamic therapy. "If necessary, I will enter their delusion, sometimes with a sense of humor," says Dr. Marotta, "but I will try to adopt a role within the delusion that can support treatment. For example I might say, 'I can accept that you are God, but then you have to accept that I am your most loyal servant and as such it is my job to care for you and bring you into the hospital.'" Does this have an immediate effect? Not necessarily. This type of conversation may take place repeatedly over weeks or months before Dr. Marotta convinces his patient to enter the hospital and begin a course of medication. This is why an enduring relationship with a provider who won't give up and continues to reach out is critical. Challenging someone's resistance requires slow and careful interaction that protects the therapeutic alliance at all costs. If a person with NBD feels they can call their doctor in a crisis, there is always hope that change can occur.

- **Communicating a "game plan" for treatment that identifies goals for success** along the way is important. One reason for resisting a diagnosis may be feelings of helplessness. If you believe that carrying a diagnosis means you are destined for a life of increasing dysfunction over which you have no control, rejecting this diagnosis may be a survival instinct. It is critical, therefore, to help someone feel they have some control over their experience. Remember Dr. Marotta's advice from Chapter Two: the more someone feels ownership of their treatment, the better. Patients need to feel that issues are solvable, and that their doctor and team will persevere until this occurs. As Dr. Marotta says:

I always acknowledge that I have the bias of a Western-trained physician. I make explicit that the role I am in is one of a hospital doctor, not, for example, a priest. This helps distinguish why I might be saying something different from what other people might have said to them that supported their delusions, culturally or otherwise. In this way, different views are respected while challenged. It all turns on trust. We, the whole team, must demonstrate that we are to be trusted, by being there and feeling the patients' suffering. This is not a communication or advertising issue. This is a human issue. We have to live with the patients in a shared community of concern, which means we are available, present, and also vulnerable. This is compassion.

- **Collaboration with family, wherever possible, should be part of the ongoing process**. Family members are also facilitators of treatment along with the team who works with their loved one. Together they form, in Dr. Marotta's words, "an extended family who share an objective, even if they don't share the same language or experience." Listening carefully and taking each other's views seriously is necessary for success. Helping a family handle the frustration that results from their loved one's denial of illness is also extremely important to the work. Shifting errors of thinking often takes a long period of time. For the staff, supporting family members during this work and helping them to support their loved one effectively is a key element in keeping treatment active and hope alive. Family members who collude in their loved one's denial of illness often feel shame as well as overwhelm. Educating a family about the reality of NBD and the possibility of successfully rebuilding a life, and helping them to find support and feel supported, is frequently necessary to combat these feelings at the heart of their resistance.

- **A doctor's and team's ability to sustain connection with someone who has NBD is critical to the patient's long-term stability and essential when dealing with someone who denies that they are ill.** What does "sustaining connection" mean, concretely? It means doctors, teams, and family members need to continue their outreach, regardless of whether or not their patient or loved one seems uninterested or uninvested in the relationship. Remember, passivity is one of the hallmarks of this disease. "With someone who is schizophrenic, you can be more connected than you are aware of because of their autism," says Dr. Marotta. "Don't interpret 'distancing' as necessarily lack of connection. You can be very central to their lives without day-to-day interaction." Try not to be defeated by lack of perceived progress. While it is important to recognize and accept the realities of your loved one's current limitations, dropping anchor while there is no wind in your sails (to continue our metaphor) does not mean that you can't continue to test the water for the emergence of currents that might help to move your ship forward.

Following Up with Andrew, Leo, and Sonia

Let's get back to our three cases. How is Dr. Marotta working with Andrew and Leo, and what can we learn from Sonia's devastating outcome? With Andrew, his current focus is on collaboration with Andrew's parents and partner, since Andrew is so repeatedly resistant. Dr. Marotta continues to pursue Andrew himself ("I won't let him escape me!") and communicates his concerns to Andrew when he reaches him, but he has accepted that for the moment Andrew is avoiding contact as much as possible. Dr. Marotta coaches Andrew's parents and partner about the importance of communicating how well they think he is doing professionally while also reminding him of past decompensation when he stopped medication. Challenging Andrew's perception that he doesn't need medication to function well is important but so is understanding that his denial of illness is fueled by grandiose defenses. Andrew needs to hear that he is doing well. If his anxiety can be calmed, then reminders that reducing medication led to past decompensations have a better chance of being heard and accepted. Dr. Marotta is encouraging Andrew's parents to urge him to continue in individual therapy, since personality issues and his grandiose defenses are significant psychological factors that fuel his denial of illness.

Dr. Marotta's focus with Leo is different. After so much time has passed in this relatively isolated holding position, he says, "The only way Leo's outlook will change is if we can pull him into a program with people who have been through what he has been through but now are succeeding." In Leo's case, Dr. Marotta sees denial of illness as a complicated mixture of biological anosognosia and the defensive need to protect himself from the enormous psychological pain that will accompany a conscious sense of what he has lost. Leo is on some medication but doesn't want to try medication that may be more effective. "A partially treated schizophrenia may in some ways be equivalent to the chronic 'haze' of an addict," says Dr. Marotta. "In this state you are not really aware of how horrible your life is, and therefore you are able to endure it."

Leo was once a tremendously promising student with enormous potential. Dr. Marotta believes that for Leo, the idea of failure, of being less than he once was, is unconsciously terrifying. "Any team that works with Leo needs to recognize that psychological fragility," says Dr. Marotta. They will need to work slowly to engender trust, and to introduce him to people who they feel will model different types of successful experience. "It is difficult to go halfway back," he notes. Most likely, Leo will need to build a different model of success for himself if he is to become less in denial and more engaged in his life. Watching others who are actively doing this is the strategy Dr. Marotta feels will be effective at this stage of Leo's life. "We need to move slowly, because to become hopeful and then not successful could be catastrophic for Leo," he muses. Patience is again at the forefront of this type of treatment.

Meanwhile, although he does not challenge Leo's denial of illness directly, he will continue to challenge his use of marijuana. Dr. Marotta strongly believes that smoking marijuana reinforces Leo's apathy and resistance to change, so he will give him repeated information and data on its problematic effect on vulnerable individuals. Sending him information is a good means of checking in with Leo. It is a useful lifeline, letting Leo know that Dr. Marotta is still around and thinking about him. Dr. Marotta also maintains contact with Leo's family and sees his support of Leo's family as critical to the work. He is honest with them about the limitations Leo may have to face, but his willingness to acknowledge the hard reality of mental illness is always balanced by his hopeful perseverance. Leo's denial of illness is a major obstacle to greater progress, but Dr. Marotta has seen The Lodge program shift the course of many "hopeless" cases. For this reason, he does not give up.

Sonia's case is an illustration of how denial of illness can be reinforced by our society's preference to diagnose other disorders over schizophrenia and schizoaffective disorders. It also illustrates the tendency of mental health providers to believe that individuals with NBD do not live smoothly functioning and meaningful lives. While the disinclination to diagnose NBD in someone who is functioning well is generally founded on good intentions, taking them off their medication can have devastating consequences. It is a fact that individuals with NBD have higher rates of death, for example, due to alcohol, drug and nicotine use, cardiovascular disease, accidents, violence and suicide.[8] Furthermore, there are only two medications known to decrease the risk for suicide in this population: lithium and clozapine.

Sonia, who had been compliant with The Lodge team's medication recommendations, was happy to stop taking her clozapine when redirected by residential staff, quickly accepting their belief that her schizoaffective diagnosis might be incorrect. Sadly, The Lodge program has worked with a number of patients whose recovery seemed similarly remarkable until they were taken off clozapine by post-Lodge program staff. "Continuing communication and collaboration between treatment teams must be a high priority," says Dr. Marotta, "if we hope to have the best possible outcomes."

LEGAL ISSUES AND DENIAL OF ILLNESS

If you don't realize that you are ill, then resistance to taking medication or hospitalization makes sense. For caretakers, however, forcing their loved one to take medication or go to the hospital may seem like the only way to help them recover. The issue of forced treatment for individuals with NBD is controversial. On one side of the argument, the antipsychiatry movement challenges the pathologizing of mental illness in general. Civil liberty advocates argue that forcing someone to be hospitalized and take medicine denies them their constitutional right to free choice. On the other side of the argument are those who believe that forced treatment for NBD is lifesaving. From this perspective, allowing someone who is psychotic and dysfunctional to go unmedicated is depriving them of their right to regain healthy brain functioning and live a full and purposeful life.

The protection of constitutional freedom for those with mental illness is federal law, but each state has the right to interpret this law as they see fit. While New York state allows limited options for treatment over objection for someone with mental illness only if they are an imminent danger to themself or others, California has just expanded this allowance to include individuals who cannot care for themselves medically or keep themselves safe. Furthermore, within each state, judges presiding over mental health courts may vary slightly in their interpretation of the law, although they are generally similar in their rulings.

Nonetheless, the reality is that throughout the United States, families are frequently prevented from getting medical treatment for their loved ones struggling with NBD if they are treatment-resistant. While our health system not only supports but encourages guardians of Alzheimer's patients, for example, to use medication to arrest the advance of increasing confusion and distorted cognitive processing in their loved ones, caretakers of confused and dysfunctional mentally ill individuals are legally discouraged from taking the same kind of action, despite overwhelming evidence that NBD is a biologically based brain illness. Even someone granted guardianship* over their loved one cannot force their loved one to take medication. Laura Brancato, JD, who specializes in mental health, guardianship, and elder law, stated this issue clearly: "[Lawyers and judges] never have the same conversation about people with Alzheimer's dementia, traumatic brain injury, even severe developmental disabilities [as we do about mental health]. We look at them in a very different way and we don't put the burden on the family member or medical facility to disprove what we believe to be true, which is that they are not thinking clearly. We certainly don't hold the medical communities or the family members [of patients with these illnesses] to the standards we hold the mental health community."[9]

Frustration and anger over this matter have prompted some families of NBD patients to threaten doctors and hospitals with lawsuits, and there is also a growing industry of individuals, titled "interventionists," who can be hired to help families deal specifically with the difficulty of their loved one refusing treatment. These mental health professionals specialize in helping families to plan interventions, which can range from meetings to address a patient's perspective to actual help accompanying a patient to a more intensive treatment setting such as a hospital or residential community. Further conversation with Ms. Brancato highlighted the following issues that arise in connection of NBD with the legal system.

---

* When an individual is declared to be "incapacitated" by the courts, they are considered incapable of controlling such things as their bank accounts, making decisions about where they live, who they visit, whether they vote, work, get married, have a driver's license and many other basic human rights. The person who is appointed by the courts to make these decisions under the prevailing law is called their guardian.

THE PROBLEM OF TIMING IN "TREATMENT OVER OBJECTION"

The legal statutes that govern "treatment over objection" vary from state to state. In New York, for example, a patient can only be treated "over objection" for two reasons: if two psychiatrists deem them a danger to self or others, or if the number of hospitalizations they have had is significant enough to indicate that the severity of their illness interferes with their ability to function. We know that early intervention in NBD is correlated with a much better recovery outcome and that putting off treatment is correlated with much more entrenched physical and psychological deterioration. Unfortunately, the legal system often obstructs early intervention because it uses the benchmark of repeated crises and hospitalizations to support a decision to medicate. If a crisis is severe enough to meet criteria for two-doctor certification (2PC), hospitalization can be mandated but limited to seventy-two hours, unless the patient continues to demonstrate severe dysfunction. If a patient is deemed not a danger to themselves or others within those seventy-two hours of medicated inpatient treatment, they can sign themselves out of the hospital.

This is the start of a "revolving door" mental health process, i.e., a patient is admitted to the hospital for a few days, released after seventy-two hours, decompensates due to lack of medication compliance, falls into a crisis necessitating rehospitalization with a 2PC for seventy-two hours, then is released to begin the process all over again. As families of loved ones know well, there is no guarantee that with each subsequent decompensation and hospitalization their loved one's response to medication will be as successful. Families are left helpless to overcome legal roadblocks to treatment, and frustrated and heartbroken knowing that with NBD the brain will continue to deteriorate over time if left untreated. Finding a lawyer who understands this fact and can urge a presiding judge to consider this issue when coming to a decision can be important.

THE PROBLEM OF COOPERATION VERSUS COERCION IN "TREATMENT OVER OBJECTION"

Individuals who are struggling with NBD are frequently paranoid and frightened. If police or fire emergency services are called to bring a loved one who is refusing treatment to a hospital, it can be traumatizing for both loved ones and their families. "A call [to emergency services] can be a very upsetting and intrusive thing," says Ms. Brancato. "[Law enforcement] actually use the same process [called extraction] as they use to get someone to come out of their jail cell in a prison facility." This can involve the use of frightening riot gear or equipment, and the trauma it causes for the patient in that moment must be treated by hospital doctors before they can deal with the patient's illness itself. Confrontations with police and the possibility of violent escalation and excessive use of force is a particularly heightened risk for people of color.[10] This type of confrontation can also cause problems for an individual post-discharge, as neighbors or landlords, fearing a repeat of this type of situation, may not want them to return. Sadly, an approximation of these types of confrontations can occur in hospitals as well. If a patient becomes violent as the result of their psychotic hallucinations and requires restraint, they and the staff can be traumatized by that experience.

Using the legal system to challenge treatment refusal can also exponentially reinforce paranoid ideas that family and providers are enemies rather than allies. Remember the heartbreaking words of one of the alum parents describing the situation with her son:

> A couple years before, I was advised I had to charge him with assault in order to get him the urgent care he needed. The police officers were the best support we had. They understood and helped me play the system as they recognized our crisis. A mother should never have to sit across from her son in a hospital court and have to say she was afraid of him in order to get him the medical attention he deserved. I don't think either one of us will ever be able to forget the pain associated with that moment. I pictured him learning to ride his bike in our cul de sac and how he trusted me to steady him until he was able to do it on his own. Our relationship was fractured. In the mental health court, while filing for conservatorship again, I was forced to list his scary symptoms and inadequacies and to recount my fears in front of him which was incredibly painful. From his perspective, I robbed him of his rights and just wanted to keep him in a locked facility. I know I hurt him terribly, and he didn't trust me again for many years.

Having others tell you what to do, especially if you feel confused and frightened, can feel punishing, controlling, and infantilizing. Ms. Brancato, in her role as a mental health lawyer, tries to facilitate a different type of experience for resistant individuals, one that involves having choices.

This is where interventionists who work under a collaborative, cooperative model can be extremely helpful. Rather than taking a coercive approach, these interventionists work to develop an alliance with resistant clients by first understanding and acknowledging their client's personal experiences and then slowly helping them to feel part of a treatment solution. Some have connections to doctors who will come to a patient in crisis to negotiate a 2PC without requiring them to go through a more traumatizing emergency room experience. If at all possible, Ms. Brancato avoids using the court system to get an individual hospitalized because its structure heightens an antagonistic dynamic.

The Problem of an Adversarial Court System

"At its core," says Ms. Brancato, "the legal process [in the United States] is an adversarial proceeding" for individuals with NBD and their families.[11] "The legal process perpetuates the idea that it's society against the person with NBD, and almost always the process is punitive. Even the documents initiating the case will usually say 'Name of the Parent' or 'Name of the Hospital" *versus* 'Name of the Person with NBD.' So, upon reading of the initial paperwork, the person with NBD already feels under attack by persons who love and care for them."

Use the legal system as sparingly as possible, Brancato advises. It can, at its best, be "a compassionate opportunity to get treatment in place," but as an aid to recovery, using the legal system is most often an uphill battle.

Dr. Marotta spoke about the changes he has noticed in the court system over the years:

> In the past, my experience of New York City judges was that they often tried to listen in detail to patient stories, make sense of the situation, and even talked to the patients to give advice. Over the last ten years there seems to be a complete emphasis on procedure and not on compassion. The appointed lawyers seem to be focused on moving cases along and not being concerned with the consequences for the patients, their families, or the communities. I am perplexed by this, and shocked when I walk the streets of New York City and pass so many suffering psychotics—overwhelmingly men—sleeping in the rain, muttering to themselves or raging at passersby. These poor people are unable to access or reject help from the

psychiatric services of our city, a city that has some of the greatest medical resources available in the world. How is it that they are left on the street, dying at a high rate from the effects of chronic disease, malnutrition, and drug use? Their lives are significantly limited and often destroyed, yet our legal system chooses to support 'autonomy' over benevolently mandated care. I am one of many voices saying our mental health system is broken. Changing the way denial of illness is treated by our legal system should be one of the facets of repair.

Where does this leave caretakers struggling to navigate the legal system in their attempts to deal with treatment resistance? The court system fails to really address the complex dynamic of NBD, Ms. Brancato admits, but although imperfect, it is the only legal system we have. So, seek out specialized help whenever possible. Find lawyers who understand the complicated issues involved in NBD recovery and have connections with collaborative support systems within the community. People are too often trapped by their sense of shame and don't ask for what they really need, she observes. Be open about the issues you face and be a persistent advocate for the needs of your loved one despite repeated challenges.

A FINAL NOTE: THE BLAME GAME

In cases of individuals whose decompensation with NBD has led to the shipwreck of difficult and sometimes terrible consequences, it is easy to play the blame game. When we don't understand and have little information to quiet our own anxiety, we point the finger, and often, sadly, that finger points unfairly at the family who, despite repeated attempts, has been unable to control the actions of their loved one. "Where was the family?" we cry. "How could they stand by and allow this to happen?" It is critical to challenge the seduction of this type of thinking and to understand that no matter how many interventions are tried, denial of illness in NBD is at times an elusive symptom, impossible to control. Of course, there are individuals with NBD whose lack of family support contributes to their decompensation, but for many others, we need to remember that family members have done everything in their power to no avail, often having been limited by the legal system we have described. Randye Kaye, in her essay "Luigi Mangione, Jordan Neely: Mental Illness in the News?

One Mother's Opinion,"[12] challenges us to remember that we rarely know the whole story. Reflecting on her situation with her own son who has slipped back into refusing treatment she says:

> So—where have we been as my son Ben faces addiction and homelessness? Right where we have been for the past two decades, ever since his diagnosis of schizophrenia:
>
> - Trying to help.
> - Trying to arrange help.
> - Fixing what we can.
> - Letting natural consequences settle—usually to no avail.
> - Setting boundaries.
> - Leaving the door open—or closing it tight if we are afraid for our safety.
> - Searching the streets.
> - Advocating for change.
> - Reaching out to each other.
> - Reversing their bad decisions.
> - Keeping young children away when our loved one is symptomatic.
> - Talking to attorneys.
> - Paying for rehab and "troubled teen" programs.
> - Declaring bankruptcy.
> - Visiting hospital and jails.
> - Educating ourselves.
> - Daring to hope.
> - Fighting with all our heart.

Denial of illness is a formidable challenge in the treatment of NBD. It is not a character flaw or a calculation. We do not blame those who receive a diagnosis of cancer or whose cancer returns after a period of remission. Let us not blame those with NBD, or their families, for the struggle to recognize and to control this difficult illness. Let us not forget that rarely in life is everything within our control.

PUTTING IT ALL TOGETHER

This chapter focuses on a topic achingly familiar to many who are dealing with the journey of NBD. Loved ones resist medication altogether, resist the most effective medication because of side effects, stop taking their medication when they feel better, or destroy their progress because they return to substance use. Denial of illness in NBD can stem from both biological and psychological causes, and carers are limited in their ability to deal with this obstacle to treatment by both legal and social constraints. It is a problem with no easy solution. But having greater clarity about the factors involved in denial of illness can impact how we approach loved ones who are struggling to feel normal. It can help us to know when and how to challenge them, or when to let go and step back. Find clinicians and specialized legal consultants with experience who can provide support and guidance. Following are some key ideas from this chapter that will be helpful to keep in mind.

KEY IDEAS FOR CHAPTER SEVEN: DENIAL OF ILLNESS

DENIAL OF ILLNESS MUST BE UNDERSTOOD FROM A BIOLOGICAL, PSYCHOLOGICAL, AND SOCIETAL PERSPECTIVE

- Biologically based **anosognosia** is one of the hallmark symptoms of NBD.

- Denial of illness can also be a **psychological defense** against the negative emotional impact of NBD for both patients and families and in support of the primacy of self and freedom.

APPROACHES TO DENIAL OF ILLNESS INCLUDE:

- establishing rapport, getting a clear diagnosis, engaging a patient in collaborative treatment, respecting the importance of medication side effects in resistance, exposing a patient to peer modeling of treatment acceptance, communicating a game plan for treatment and recovery, collaborating with family, and sustaining outreach regardless of patient response.

LEGAL ISSUES RELATED TO DENIAL OF ILLNESS:

- the problem of timing in "treating over objection"
- the problem of cooperation versus coercion in "treating over objection"

- the problem of an adversarial court system

- use of specialized help, including mental health lawyers and collaborative interventionists

Chapter 8

SAFE HARBORS

"Our son is on the road to his best self. He is still living with serious
mental illness. But we have always hoped he would have purpose
in his life as well as joy and to know he is loved. He is smiling again
and so are we."

—*Alum Parent*

Charlie is away at a full-time graduate program. Leslie is living in a step-
down community, taking classes and working part-time. Stuart is living on
his own and enjoying city life. Bernice has finished graduate school and is
working at a well-paying job. Matthew is living in a small residential community and making furniture. Jimmy is living independently and working
part-time at a job in a suburban town, planning to start taking classes. Bernice has a boyfriend. Stuart loves his support group. Jonathan, William,
and Charlie enjoy a continuing friendship. What is a "best life"? Each of
these individuals would answer this question differently and has journeyed
a long, difficult road to get there.

Aligning intellectual capacity, aspirations, ability to sustain concentration, and ability to respond adaptively to stress can be frustrating and
demoralizing to someone who wants a satisfying and independent life but
whose existence has been impacted by repeated and disorganizing psychotic symptoms. Charlie, Leslie, Stuart, Bernice, Matthew, Jimmy, Jonathan, and William have all had sustained relationships with staff who

have helped them to define personal satisfaction and create evolving goals. From the perspective of The Lodge team, a best life is never dependent on attaining a certain level of achievement, but it does involve feeling empowered, being able to find a sense of belonging and engagement in one's life. If you believe, as Dr. Marotta and The Lodge team do, that remaining in a psychotic state is not living a "best" life, there are many factors involved in finding greater happiness and sustaining recovery. Part of the magic of sustained connection to a doctor and team is that they know your history and can help you to integrate the different aspects of your life.

Coming to terms with the continuing impact that vulnerability to brain dysregulation will play in your life is an enormous challenge. It means accepting that coping with NBD is a lifetime voyage, not a journey to a single destination. The team believes that post-discharge, patients still need support to solidify their understanding of medication's importance in their sustained stability. They also need a less structured (supervised) but safe environment in which to practice a more engaged life. They need time to gain confidence in themselves, to become more self-directed and anchored in the routines of daily life. They need to practice and enjoy connection to others.

DISCHARGE PLANNING: BUILDING A MEANINGFUL LIFE

The mission of The Lodge team is to stay open to the experience and needs of their patients. It is to chart a new recovery process and, when the time comes, help them to find a safe harbor where the next leg of the voyage can continue. The seeds of discharge planning are planted in the very beginning of a Lodge stay, when families are educated about The Lodge program and what will come after. Jackie Ordoñez states it succinctly: "Historically, ninety percent of our patients do not go home after their stay at The Lodge. We don't have all the facilities for them to really practice life. That's what they do when they go to a long-term step-down program."

The average length of stay for a patient at The Lodge is six weeks to three months. How a family responds to the idea of transitioning to a different vessel (often a longer-term residential experience) once their loved one is discharged from The Lodge has a direct influence on how discharge planning is handled. Families have different travel ideas and different budgets. Whatever fantasies they have had about their loved one's life following discharge from The Lodge, they will now have more concrete recommendations to think about. They need time to process the information and decide what works best for them. For some, education about longer-term placements will prove comforting. For others, it creates anxiety. The team listens. They know a lot can happen during a resident's stay to influence a family's orientation toward discharge options. For this reason, residents are not themselves involved in discharge planning in the early stages. They are protected from any information that might be further destabilizing or collude with their resistance. The team wants their focus to remain in the present.

Social workers at The Lodge are the primary discharge planners, but some psychiatrists enjoy collaborating in this process, and this is often helpful, especially if families are hesitant or need convincing. "I can tell the parents why we think [discharge plans] are so important. But at the end of the day the parents are key to the decision," says Ordoñez. If a family is not fully on board with discharge plans, chances are high their loved one will resist them too. If a resident's primary social worker and psychiatrist talk to the family together, it lends weight to the recommendations and helps them to understand that discharge decisions are team-based. This is an important message. Family consultants may also be involved in discharge planning, and the most successful outcomes are smooth collaborations between all involved. Everyone's goal is the same: finding a place where a resident can continue to be supported on medication with the addition of program structures that offer increasing levels of independence and community involvement.

Toward the end of a resident's stay, planning will build momentum. Recommendations given to the family will have already been discussed, concerns ironed out, or plans redesigned if necessary. Residents are now brought into the process. Their acceptance of the plan is necessary; enthusiasm at this stage is not required, as the team knows that change is anxiety-producing, even if a resident feels they are ready to leave The Lodge. If a resident is hesitant, speaking on the phone to the head of a recommended program is sometimes helpful, and on rare occasions a visit to the program may occur. If a resident is not discharged to a residential program, the team will work hard to make sure as many support structures as possible are in place wherever they go.

At The Lodge, discharge planning is heavily influenced by the belief that continuing on prescribed medications is essential to sustaining and augmenting gains made in the program. Each resident leaves the program with a finely titrated medication regimen. Residents are different in their degree of medication compliance, however. Some are relatively happy to continue medication when they leave and can thrive in programs that focus on more patient-driven treatment. Others are ready to get off the medication boat completely the minute they leave The Lodge program, believing their journey is totally finished. As previously discussed, this is enormously risky, and the team prefers to discharge these patients to a program that will support The Lodge team's medication recommendations. Collaborations with residential program directors are particularly helpful when a resident or their family is ambivalent about discharge plans and needs additional persuading or support to tolerate the transition to a new stage of treatment.

How does the team know when a resident is ready for discharge? This is a difficult question to answer because there are no exact outcome measures. The best answer is that the team is looking at a resident's transformation. They are reviewing what their abilities were before their psychotic illness began, they are assessing how the psychotic illness has transformed their functioning, they are evaluating their response to medications while in the program, and they are monitoring the degree of their return to pre-psychotic functioning. If discharge is not triggered prematurely, all of these factors are weighed relative to one another, with the addition of financial factors, and go into the decision about discharge readiness. Readiness to leave the program does not mean that transformation is at an end. It means that a resident has achieved a level of stability and functioning that will support their life in a less structured environment.

It is important to understand, having a stable life "[is] not about doing great all the time," says Dr. Brown, one of the team's former senior psychiatrists, who continues to work with some discharged Lodge patients in her private practice. "It's always about how you deal with adversity when it happens. Because adversity is inevitable. So in the program, we figure out a way to introduce that adversity when it's the right time or when the person can actually cope with it." Preparing a resident to become better able to deal with change and adversity while they are in the program is preparation for life when they leave The Lodge. Handling everyday stressors without decompensating is a necessary prerequisite for everyday experience. "I think the process of the illness actually creates rigidity," adds Dr. Brown. "And then to soften that rigidity and create flexibility.... it just takes a ton of time, and you have to stay with it." A resident is ready for discharge when they can adjust to stressful moments, can connect with others, and can follow the guidance of trusted support staff. Over time, with growing understanding about how to manage their illness, many Lodge alums go back to school or settle into a life that involves some kind of purposeful work and connection to others.

Transformation takes time, and therefore staff resist early predictions of what the ultimate outcome for a resident may be. At every stage of a resident's Lodge program voyage, the team is assessing how much the patient can handle, what they find motivating, and what they will need to progress toward this vision of a meaningful life. One resident is happiest when he is surrounded by nature and the more peaceful existence of rural life. Another resident craves knowledge and the stimulation of going to school. And yet another feels more empowered by having a job. For some, living back at home with their family grants a sense of safety and well-being. For others, satisfaction stems from living on their own. Landing in a place which will help these experiences to flourish is the next step after discharge from The Lodge program.

Assessing what level of care a resident will continue to need, how medication-compliant they will be, what their family can afford and what the state will contribute, and what the resident wants are sometimes difficult factors to align, and the team may have to work hard to sell a program or effect a compromise. Some people will go back to families or temporary step-down houses after discharge and eventually go on to lead fully independent lives. Others may, after years of hospitalizations, need longer-term assisted living for an indefinite period of time. It is clear, however, that sustained recovery following discharge from The Lodge requires supportive structures to be in place.

POST-DISCHARGE SUPPORT STRUCTURES

The following is an overview of post-discharge support structures. It is not meant to be comprehensive but rather a snapshot of the types of support structures a patient might transition to when they leave an inpatient-based program.

Psychiatric Care

Since medication and medication adjustment are so central to a sustained recovery, patients and their families dealing with NBD need to maintain a strong relationship with a psychiatrist after they are discharged from The Lodge. Many who continue to live locally, and even some who move farther away, continue to see Lodge psychiatrists, all of whom have outpatient practices. If a patient needs alternative psychiatric care, The Lodge team tries to help them find it, and if a patient is discharged to a residential community, their psychiatric care may be transitioned there. Even so, families and patients have often developed strong, trusting relationships with their Lodge psychiatrists during their stay in the program, and it is not unusual for them to check back periodically for guidance or just to update them on how life is going since discharge.

What is the nature of a continuing psychiatric relationship? Like an individual with diabetes who maintains a long-standing relationship with their endocrinologist or primary care physician, a person with NBD will similarly benefit from an enduring relationship with a psychiatrist they trust. In moments of crisis, they may see their psychiatrist more frequently. In times of stability, they may require only periodic check-ins. The goal of this relationship is to help a person maintain not only stable but optimal functioning. This means making sure voices don't return and delusions don't reappear. It means monitoring a person's ability to handle stress and adversity and adjusting medication accordingly. It means having a sense of a person's life and daily functioning so that upheavals don't go unnoticed.

Unlike a more traditional therapeutic alliance, the shape of the relationship depends on what will help a person feel most connected and supported. Dr. Brown builds with Legos with one patient, who finds face-to-face conversation difficult. She trades pictures of pets with another, so he feels connected and knows she is "thinking of him." Dr. Marotta often teases or jokes with his patients as a way of connecting. He welcomes their calls when they are away, shares ideas about school projects, listens to stories of personal successes and perceived failures, and gives direct advice if he is worried about their behavior. Parents are also welcome to call him. Effectively supporting your loved one with NBD often requires decisions about handling moments of destabilization or making choices about when to step in or back away. Dr. Marotta, like the other Lodge psychiatrists, is always available to talk things over. Having the ability to reach out to your doctor without making an appointment can mean the difference between overwhelm and the ability to tolerate and navigate a difficult situation. Relationships between patients, their families, and trusted mental health professionals often last for decades.

INDIVIDUAL THERAPY

Especially in the early stages after discharge, it is helpful for someone with NBD to have a therapist who helps them to cope with the stresses of everyday life. If they have gone to a residential setting that includes clinical services, that help will be provided there. If they are in step-down housing that has no programming or are back with their family, some form of individual therapy should be added on if possible.

Some residents continue to see their psychiatrist for both medication monitoring and individual psychotherapy following discharge. Other residents work with an individual therapist, sometimes the social worker they saw at The Lodge, in addition to a psychiatrist. In the latter case, collaboration between the psychiatrist and therapist is key to understanding a fuller picture of functioning. Therapists who are more involved in monitoring the flow of a patient's daily life can give important feedback to the psychiatrist, who is deciding whether or not a medication dosage is working or if a medication needs to be changed or combined with something else. Ideally, families or patient companions* are also involved in this feedback loop. They see patients in the context of family dynamics or daily routines, which are important additional markers of functioning. Collaborative information supports early intervention if destabilization begins to occur. The more a patient learns to identify early indicators of difficulty themselves, the more they will be able to take control, reach out if necessary, and chart the course of their own life.

RESIDENTIAL SETTINGS/THERAPEUTIC FARMS

As is reflected in the history of SHH, the tradition of bringing patients to heal in peaceful settings has a long legacy. While there are certainly urban

---

* Some families hire a "companion" to live with or accompany their loved one during daily routines.

residential communities, many therapeutic communities are located in more rural settings, where there is less stimulation and less exposure to more typically urban problems like drug use. This type of residential experience was pioneered by individuals like Virgil Stucker,* whose life over the past several decades has been dedicated to the development of creative therapeutic communities. These programs can be relatively short (one to six months) or long-term (six months to years), often include clinical services, and may involve a work component (for example, helping to harvest maple syrup, bake bread, make furniture). The success of work-based programs is predicated on the idea that working and contributing to the welfare of a community builds self-esteem, pride, and a sense of accomplishment.[1]

Dr. Marotta agrees: "To be able to do something you feel good about and to be able to maintain social relationships is at the heart of a meaningful life." Contributing is not dependent on a certain level of ability. One person may count eggs for the bread the bakery is baking, another can work independently to build furniture for the community, a third may enjoy harvesting vegetables from the farm. Each activity requires a different level of attention and focus and different needs for supervision and abstract planning. While forms of participation may evolve over the course of a person's stay in a program, the goal of these activities remains the same: to support empathic connection to others while building an individual's sense of purpose and self-worth.

The development of interpersonal skills and a sense of personal self-confidence is at the heart of all residential programs. **Therapeutic Farms** are a subset of residential communities that approach these goals through therapeutic farming. Farming and gardening, helping with animals, and working the tasks necessary to sustain an organic farm community provide many therapeutic benefits. As with all work-based programs, activities vary in the degree of independence and supervision they require, but living on the farm generally involves teamwork, skills training, and problem-solving. Therapeutic farms and more rural residential settings are a particularly good match for individuals who are drawn to the natural world and the peace you can find working the land.

---

* Virgil Stucker was the founding Executive Director of the CooperRiis Healing Community. He has served as founding board member of several healing communities and has served as the executive director and president of seven not-for-profit organizations. He has been a leader in this field with over forty years of experience, focusing on the healing power of community, creativity, and philanthropy.

Urban residential programs generally place their residents in supervised apartments but require group participation to encourage social experience and teamwork. They structure activities and clinical services throughout each day, increasing an individual's level of independent functioning as they prove able to sustain recovery behavior. Going back to school or beginning to work at a job is integrated into the program at more advanced levels of independence, as is living with check-in accountability but less overall supervision. Individuals who are at higher levels of functioning often mentor those who are newer in the program.

SAFE HOUSES/STEP-DOWN HOUSING/GROUP HOMES

Step-down housing is housing that provides some degree of supervision and assistance to individuals who are discharged from the hospital, but few, if any, programmatic services. While all step-down housing encourages residents to be substance-free, some houses are specifically designated for sober living and may be affiliated with associations like AA or NA. If a resident is going to transfer to step-down housing or a group home, The Lodge team tries to make sure that additional supportive structures are in place. This means making sure individual therapy and psychiatric care continue, helping to develop a connection to local AA or NA groups if appropriate, and facilitating activities like going to the gym, pursuing a hobby, or working part-time in a local business.

In step-down housing, there is always someone present at the house to assist residents with taking their medication and other activities of daily living. Programs vary in the degree to which they offer residents other forms of assistance (help to coordinate clinical care, rides to appointments, tutoring services, meal services, laundry assistance, etc.). Similar to residential housing, there is a diversity in length of stay in step-down housing. However, many individuals stay longer in step-down housing, as they are becoming integrated into the community and more independent during this period.

SUPPORT GROUPS

Support for patients and families who are struggling with NBD is of utmost importance in their treatment journey. What follows is an overview of a few of the available support structures, organizations, online and in-person groups, books, and podcasts. Please note that these are only a few specific examples, reflective of the array of resources available.

Families who are struggling with NBD and related addiction issues can find valuable educational resources and links to support group networks for both patients and family members in national and online programs like the **National Alliance of Mental Illness, Depression and Bipolar Support Alliance, Alcoholics Anonymous, Assertive Community Treatment, and Smart Recovery.** These types of groups and educational experiences are often peer-led or self-directed, some following a preset structure and training for peer group leaders, and others more open-ended, focused on sharing personal experiences.

The National Alliance on Mental Illness (www.nami.org), in particular, can be a tremendous support for family members as they struggle to find their way through this evolving experience. NAMI's website states it is the nation's largest grassroots organization "dedicated to building better lives for the millions of Americans affected by mental illness."[2] Founded in 1979, it now has affiliate organizations in every state. The organization includes educational components, structured peer-led support groups for both family members and patients, advocacy, and forums for sharing personal stories. There are links to a wide variety of resources, and when you are in the midst of confusion and overwhelm, NAMI support services can be an invaluable lifeline in complement to psychiatric and other support structures.

One such support structure is **Team Daniel Running for Recovery** (teamdanielrunningforrecovery.org), a good example of how a specialized community-based program, accessible to a wide range of families, can provide life-affirming support. Team Daniel was founded by Robert Laitman, MD, and his wife Ann Mandel Laitman, MD, in response to their struggles to find appropriate treatment for their son Daniel, who had developed a resistant psychotic disorder. The program is dedicated to using clozapine to treat individuals with NBD. Based on their own research on clozapine's superior effectiveness with resistant psychosis, and unable to find a psychiatrist willing to start their son on this medication, the Laitmans began their own clozapine-based program, with enormous success. Based in Westchester, NY, Dr. Laitman and his team prescribe clozapine for a large group of patients, who the Laitmans continue to follow themselves. Support for patients revolves around a weekly running group led by Dr. Laitman, a serious runner, and weekly family gatherings. Team Daniel welcomes anyone in the larger community who believes in the efficacy of clozapine to join their online weekly Zoom support group meetings, as well as to become a member of their private Facebook group, which has over 5,000 members nationally and globally. Clozapine is seen as the key to NBD long-term stability, and programmatic suggestions (including running to combat weight gain, and various supplements to deal with fatigue and other side effects) have been developed to complement medication intervention. Currently, Team Daniel involves two equally important components: one, political outreach to support the early use of clozapine in the treatment of schizophrenia and promote necessary changes in regulations surrounding its use; and two, enormous support for patients and families, who gain strength and hope from shared experiences. For those parents who feel empowered by taking action, there is an associated group, The Angry Moms, who work with the Laitmans to effect systemic change. For others, the simple act of gathering with people who understand their struggles is part of a healing process. The Team Daniel website offers valuable links to other resources. The Lodge has referred many patients to Team Daniel, and wherever possible, works collaboratively with this organization.

Another significant resource is the **CureSZ Foundation** (curesz. org), located in Cincinnati, Ohio. CureSZ provides advocacy, information, advice, and educational and supportive resources to enhance the understanding of schizophrenia as a treatable neuropsychiatric illness.

The **STEP Learning Collaborative** (ctearlypsychosisnetwork.org), a collaboration between the Connecticut Department of Mental Health & Addiction Services and Yale University Department of Psychiatry, was created to "build a system of care for recent onset schizophrenia across Connecticut." While its services are primarily based in Connecticut, they provide educational webinars, family workshops, skills trainings, and consultations to the general public, as well as to providers.

Books/Podcasts about Personal Experience

Hearing about someone else's experience can sometimes be a lifesaver, a buoy thrown out by a fellow passenger who is no longer actively drowning themselves. Especially in the beginning of this journey, there is a lot of information to take in, and it is easy to become overwhelmed and feel that you are alone in your struggle. Additionally, there is often a disconnect between what is needed and what is available for those struggling with NBD. Putting together the necessary structures to support and then sustain your loved one's recovery journey requires energy, perseverance, and advocacy. It requires learning and understanding the system, and families who are further along in this process often have valuable, compassionate guidance to share. Please see the section following the Appendix for some examples of the many books and podcasts which are invaluable resources in this regard.

PUTTING IT ALL TOGETHER

We know that it is scary to leave a familiar vessel, whether it is an institution, a home, or an out-patient experience. If you have reached this place in your journey, our hope is that it is because you or your loved one have achieved a level of stability and are ready for the next step. This is a time of transition and vulnerability, but also of hope and anticipation. Having a solid, well-thought-out plan for next steps is critical, and the following key ideas can guide you. This plan, once a loved one is discharged from the hospital, is critically important if gains made during an inpatient stay are to be maintained. It is important to remember that NBD is a chronic illness. Stability is to be fiercely guarded, because each time an individual relapses it places enormous stress on a vulnerable system. We understand that the post-hospital options for individuals with NBD may be limited by factors including finances, geography, and family dynamics. We offer the resources in this book to help you do the best you can. Build in support structures that include a stable psychiatric team and community allies well-versed in the nature of this chronic disease.

KEY IDEAS FOR CHAPTER EIGHT:
SAFE HARBORS

Coping with NBD is a lifetime voyage with different safe harbors along the way. When a hospital program experience ends, it is not the end of the journey. Discharge planning is critical to continuing recovery.

- **Discharge planning is a process**. It begins with education about possible options and involves aligning the needs of the patient, the family's perspective and finances, and understanding what financial aid might be available. It works best if team members collaborate.

- **Patients should not be distracted by early discharge planning**.

- **Different options include:** urban or rural residential settings, step-down houses or group homes, and moving back with family or into supervised apartment life.

- **Programs that support medication compliance are optimal.**

- **Post-discharge structures can vary widely, but all patients need the following support**: medication management, help with the structure of daily living, help with sobriety, community connection and support groups, help engaging in some form of school or work.

- **Families need continued connection to providers and support communities**. The ability to connect with providers outside regular appointments can help families navigate turbulence; examples include support groups such as NAMI's Family to Family, podcasts, and books that help family members feel less isolated in their experience. References for these are provided above in this chapter.

Thoughts from a Couple
of Our Alums

Here are some honest thoughts from two of our alums about aspects of their Lodge experience, as they progressed from the extended stay phase to discharge and life outside the hospital.

Q: What were the most important things about your Lodge experience?

A: *"One of the most important things was that I was around people that were going through similar issues."*

"I think the most important aspects were the time away from home, the doctors, the program, and the overall living experience. The most important aspects of my time at The Lodge were the other patients and the nurses. The other patients gave me a sense of community, a feeling that I wasn't alone in my mental health journey. The nurses gave me a feeling of safety, knowing if I had any sort of problem, I could go and talk to them whenever I needed. Also the general atmosphere of Silver Hill, the beautiful grounds, the good food, and overall therapeutic nature of the hospital were all important to my recovery."

Q: How was it different from other hospitalizations?

A: *"I don't have much experience in other hospitalizations. I only went to one other hospital before Silver Hill and was only there for a few hours. That being said, the experience was completely different. The hospital put me in a gown and assigned me to a room. The room had one twin bed in it and nothing else. I felt unsafe and trapped in this hospital. It was the complete opposite of Silver Hill. At Silver Hill I felt safe, cared for, and felt like I belonged."*

"Silver Hill was my first and only hospitalization so I can't speak to experiences at other hospitals."

Q: How important is length of stay to getting better?

A: *"I'm not sure if it was the length of stay that was important or the fact that I trusted what my team thought was the best to be important. If you guys had told me that I needed to extend even more I would have trusted that that was what was best and vice versa."*

"While during my stay I was upset I was asked to stay for more than a month, I think the fact I stayed for longer actually made all the difference in my long-term mental health. Becoming healthy takes time. I think if one rushes their treatment,

Continued ➤

they are so much more likely to end up back in the hospital in their future. I would highly recommend to any of my peers to stay longer than they feel necessary, as in the long run it will be worth it."

Q: Did you make any friends while you were in the program?

A: *"Absolutely. I made a lot of friends. Whether it was pick-up basketball or watching movies or playing board games at the house, I always felt comforted by my friends at Silver Hill. When I first arrived at Silver Hill, I was extremely lonely. My mental health struggles severed all my relationships with others. But after a few weeks at Silver Hill, the friends I made helped me out of that difficult time."*

"I felt like I made friends but didn't keep in touch after I was discharged."

Q: Would you go back to The Lodge if you needed to?

A: *"Yes, I would."*

"Absolutely I would. That being said, I've been consistently healthy, performing well in school, and happy since Silver Hill and I hope to never have to be hospitalized again."

Q: Has your view of doctors and therapists changed? If so, why?

A: *"Before Silver Hill I talked to a therapist weekly but was skeptical of psychiatrists and medicine overall. Now my views have changed. The medicine I'm now taking has had a tremendously positive impact on my life and I trust my doctors fully. My doctors and therapists have supported me and kept me stable, and I am now so grateful for their influence in my life."*

"Kind of. I think I also have a unique perspective after working [with doctors myself]...."

Q: What medicines do you take?

A: *"I take clozapine, Lamictal, oxytocin, and Ritalin."*

"I take clozapine in the evening and Nuvigil with oxytocin in the morning."

Q: What do you think are the most helpful medicines?

A: *"I think the clozapine is the most helpful medicine. Once I started taking clozapine, I felt like I was truly recovering. I believe the medication has been responsible for my overall stability."*

"I think that Lamictal and clozapine are probably the most helpful."

Q: If you are taking oxytocin, how do you think it helps you?

Continued ➤

A: *"I'm not sure how oxytocin helps me."*

"Oxytocin is the only medicine that I don't take consistently. I've gone through periods of taking it and not taking it. Currently I've been taking it consistently for a couple of months and the most noticeable difference is a kind of warm feeling that I have."

Q: What persuaded you to take your medicines if you were initially resistant?

A: *"I wasn't initially resistant to taking medication. I was sick and wanted to get better. There had been periods of time when I wanted to see if I could wean off, and with the clozapine it got to a certain point where I really wanted to see if I could get off of it. But I could see after I got below a certain point that I needed to go back up at least a little bit, and I haven't tried to drop since."*

"I was initially resistant but wasn't once it became clear to me that I was not well. It took a long time to realize this. My desire to be healthy again made me realize the right path was to start taking medication."

Q: How difficult is it to stay on medicine after being discharged? If it is difficult, what helps you to take it?

A: *"It has not been difficult for me to stay on the medicine. I have never even thought of getting off it. I want to stay healthy and therefore I take my meds."*

"The only hard part about staying on my medication is that I feel like my life kind of revolves around the clozapine. If I have friends in town, I can't take the clozapine before I go out because then I will get tired. But then if I decide to go out and not take it till I get back in, I'm going to be asleep till 4:00 p.m., and I've found that I'm really sensitive when I don't take it at all. So, as I said, it kind of feels like my life revolves around it in some ways."

Q: What are the side effects of your medicines and how bad are the side effects?

A: *"The most notable side effect for me is the fatigue from clozapine. I sleep for probably an average of ten hours a night, and it's manageable but it does feel like I have to make plans around when I take my clozapine. Also, I have gained about fifty pounds since I was prescribed clozapine—I was also borderline underweight when I started—but exercise has helped me keep it in check and I try to generally only eat when I'm hungry."*

"Some general side effects have been feeling hungry constantly and becoming slightly obsessive. But I've now learned to eat healthy in ways I never had to before, and I

Continued ➤

try to look at the OCD as positive. It helps me stay focused in school. The only side effect that really has brought me trouble over the past few years is akathisia. That being said, recently I have rarely experienced it. But every once in a while I'll take my medicine and about forty minutes later I'll have an extremely uncomfortable sensation that almost mimics intense anxiety. When in this state it's nearly impossible to lie down and I have to keep walking. I've learned over the years that when this happens I can take Benadryl, which kicks in in about a half hour, I can take a cold shower, or I can get sick. I've noticed akathisia is more likely to occur when I've eaten sugar in the evening."

Q: What helped you cope with side effects? The staff? Other medications? Stoicism?

A: *"Speaking with my doctor and therapists has helped overall. For the hunger I've found a diet that requires me to weigh myself daily which helps me not overeat. For the OCD, you just try to look at it as a positive. And for akathisia, the methods listed above help me with my side effects."*

"I think acceptance has helped me, and I don't think that I have had very many side effects."

Q: Where did you go when you left the hospital?

A: *"When I left the hospital, Covid lock-down was just beginning so I went back and stayed with my family for the summer. And then moved and began attending community college."*

"After Silver Hill I went back to the outpatient program in my city. But then after a few months, Covid hit and I left the city to live with my parents and continued this same outpatient program virtually."

Q: Was your discharge plan a good one? If yes, why? If not, why?

A: *"I honestly don't remember my discharge plan very well. I was supposed to go to a farm but because of Covid it fell through, and I was released to my family. Silver Hill helped me to find a doctor where I was living, and I continued to work with my social worker from Silver Hill."*

"I think my discharge plan ended up to be great. I didn't want to go to my placement at first, but it ended up being the right place for me. The people there, both patients and staff, gave me a community which helped me settle back into the real world. I could continue my life while still attending therapy groups. Even when I enrolled back in school I still attended various groups such as 'men's process,' 'relationship group,' and a book club."

Continued ➤

Q: Have you made friends since you have left the hospital?

A: *"Since leaving the hospital I haven't made very many friends. It's probably been one of the things that I've struggled with the most since discharge."*

"I have made a few, but to be honest this is an area in my life I hope to develop in the future. I have been so focused on my studies and therefore have not had a very lively social life. That being said, I've become way closer to my family. My brother and I speak all the time...and my mom, dad, and I are very close. I've even gotten closer to my cousins and grandparents."

Q: Have you been able to do something that makes you happy? School? Work? Hobby?

A: *"School and reading have been good for me. I've recently found out that I like putting things together as well, so that's kind of a hobby. I think that using my brain and getting out of the house has been a big part of my recovery."*

"Absolutely. I've been happier these past few years than I ever have been. I've been fully immersed in my classes; I exercise consistently and spend the rest of my free time doing things I love to do."

Q: Do you think staying on your medicine is important to your health and happiness?

A: *"Of course. I think, in a sense, good health is happiness, and I have no intentions to get off my medication any time soon."*

"I think that it's important to my health, which is important to my happiness. I don't think being on my medication is stopping me from being happy anymore."

Q: Do you think staying sober is important to your health and happiness? If not, what and how much do you use?

A: *"I think that staying off of drugs has been very important to my health and happiness. I still drink but I haven't smoked weed or done any other drugs since I was admitted to the hospital several years ago."*

"Of course. I've been sober for seven years now and haven't even had alcohol in the past four years. I don't smoke cigarettes either and I don't even crave any of those vices anymore. Over time I just realized that drugs and alcohol didn't actually make me happier or healthier, so I put them down. Being sober has helped me accomplish many of my goals."

Q: Who do you rely on for support? Has your relationship with your family changed?

Continued ➤

A: *"Absolutely. When I was at my peak of unhealthiness I didn't even speak to any of my family. Now I'm so close with all of them. I rely on my family, as well as my therapist and doctor too."*

"I mostly rely on my family for support. My mom and dad, they've seen how committed I've been to recovery, so it's made things easier between us and they trust me a lot more. It's also been a good gauge for my progress."

Q: Do you have a spiritual life? Has this changed since your hospitalization?

A: *"I'm very much not spiritual or religious. This was the case before and after my hospitalization. I understand why being religious or spiritual could be really important to people though."*

"Not necessarily a spiritual life, but since hospitalization I've come up with a list of activities that support my mental health. I do yoga twice a week, fitness with a trainer twice a week, I run a few times a week, and lift weights alone. I swim every once in a while. I do breathing exercises, I meditate, and I stick to a healthy diet. I read, write, and confide in my therapists and doctors. All these activities have become my spiritual life."

Chapter 9

Navigating Your Own Waterways: Key Channel Markers to Guide Your Journey

Disparity in accessing the kind of treatment that occurs in The Lodge program is one of the failures of our mental health system. Further research and advocacy are necessary to drive larger-scale changes to mental health delivery and treatment, but the mission of the Center for the Treatment and Study of Neuropsychiatric Disorders is to try, on a smaller scale, to reach a wider diversity of patients. Partnering with individuals and institutions wherever possible, educational initiatives and research based on Lodge program outcomes are already informing the work being done with a wider range of NBD patients in more diverse settings.

Our hope is that the information presented within these pages, with the lessons learned from the work of Dr. Marotta and The Lodge program team, can support you on your individual journey. Broadly speaking, these lessons fall into the following areas:

- the critical importance of enduring connection with providers

- addressing constellations of symptoms versus unitary diagnostic categories

- the central role of individualized medication regimens, sobriety, and a calm environment to sustained recovery

- the importance of creating a collaborative treatment experience for patients and families

- the importance of time and patience in sustaining recovery

- the importance of developing a patient's sense of agency and relationship to their family and community

Most importantly, we believe connection is at the hub of change. Healing is not merely a function of specific technical skills and chemical formulas but emerges from the building and sustaining of long-term relationships between patients, families, and clinicians. Clinicians who are willing to do this, to extend lifelines whenever they are needed and to remind patients and families to never give up, are worth searching for. These are the passionate clinicians who have the ability to acknowledge and manage the reality of limited functioning in the present moment while maintaining a belief that future functioning can be significantly improved. They are anchored by both their honesty and their hope, and patients and families need both.

The staff at The Lodge are committed to the mission of rebuilding lives torn apart by NBD, and there is no doubt that an extended stay in The Lodge program helps them to persevere successfully. But the power of connection can take place anywhere. There are numerous individuals, agencies, programs, and institutions (other captains, crews, and vessels) to be found outside of The Lodge experience that can play a role in providing help, guidance, and resources to those suffering from NBD. For example, members of assertive community treatment (ACT) teams, residential setting staff, or visiting community mental health workers, among others, can all be powerful agents of change. We recognize that frustration and overwhelm often feel insurmountable to patients and families sloughing through the numerous obstacles in the path of recovery. But it only takes one person to make the experience of this journey feel different and bearable. Keep searching if you have not found them already.

Ideally, there will be a core group of providers that works together for an extended period of time to help an individual regain their potential. If you are still in the process of assembling the team you hope to work with, the following template of questions is designed to help you. Listening to the answers to these questions, or questions you devise of a similar nature, should shine a spotlight on individuals engaged in the kind of committed and collaborative treatment that we believe all NBD patients and their families deserve. They are based on the lessons presented in this book, reflecting an approach which has helped many patients move from despair to a meaningful life they never thought possible. We do not underestimate the difficulty of this task or how many times you may feel like giving up. But please, take our words to heart. Rebuilding a life ravaged by NBD is possible. Let hope be the wind in your sails.

Ask these Questions/ Champion these Goals!

Questions for Carers to Ask of Treatment Programs

What criteria do you use for a successful outcome of treatment?
> Seek providers who believe someone with NBD can eventually feel connected to others, can have a sense of agency through work or hobbies, and can feel that their life has meaning.

How long do you ideally work with your patients?
> Seek providers who value and work to maintain long-term relationships with their patients.

How do you/your team maintain contact with your patients?
> Seek providers who are willing to reach out to their patients, not just wait for patients to call or come to them.

Does your evaluation involve a physical work-up?
> Seek providers who believe that ruling in or out medical issues is critical to understanding the problem and minimizing errors and will collaborate with consultants who have specialized expertise if necessary. Seek someone who is willing to argue with the insurance company to support necessary evaluations.

How closely do you work with family members?

Find providers who believe their relationship to their patient's family is critical to treatment and are willing to coach family members through crises. Look for providers who demonstrate a sensitivity to and consideration of systemic and cultural issues, as well as individual family dynamics.

How do you handle anosognosia?

Seek providers who work to develop trust with their patients, who focus on helping with issues beyond diagnosis, and who believe in maintaining contact even if their patient is not following directions.

How do you handle relapse?

Seek providers who continue to reach out to their patients and who also maintain contact with family members in an effort to reestablish a lifeline to treatment. Seek a clinician who is willing to rethink a treatment plan if necessary.

How important is sobriety to long-term stability?

Seek providers who strongly promote sobriety as important to long-term stability. In some cases, substance use may need to be treated as a separate issue, but it is generally a significant impediment to recovering full potential.

How do you handle medication side effects?

Seek providers who understand the validity of patient complaints and are willing to partner with their patients to minimize side effects while reminding them of the potential benefits if they push through initial difficulties.

What medications do you use? Are you willing to prescribe clozapine?

Seek providers who are willing to use a variety of medications, including clozapine. Find someone who is willing to address constellations of symptoms versus a single diagnosis.

How do you handle negative symptoms? Would you be willing to try oxytocin?

Find providers who recognize that negative symptoms are a central factor in patients' inability to live meaningful lives and are willing to try a variety of medications and other strategies to minimize these symptoms.

What do you see as the goal of treatment?

Seek providers who strive to help their patients reintegrate into their community, rebuild a sense of identity, and fulfill their dreams in some fashion.

QUESTIONS FOR CARERS TO ASK
RESIDENTIAL SETTINGS

Is there a community component to your setting? If so, in what ways does the community come together?

Seek a setting where there is as strong a component of peer support and peer modeling as possible.

What is your setting's philosophy about sobriety and NBD?

Seek a setting where the importance of sobriety is stressed and repeatedly encouraged; understand, however, that complete sobriety is challenging to maintain in our society.

What is your setting's philosophy about medication compliance and NBD?

Seek a setting where medication compliance is strongly encouraged and facilitated through work with peer groups and close contact with staff and families. Ask if the program has a history of changing treatment plans that are working based on their "ideology," e.g., taking someone off of medication who has achieved stability because they are doing so well.

How much education about NBD and drug use is provided? How is this accomplished?

Seek a setting that believes in the importance of education about a wide variety of topics related to recovery from NBD. Ideally, education comes both from staff and from peer mentoring.

How are residents encouraged to develop a sense of personal agency?

Find a setting that offers the opportunity for residents to participate in team-based skill development and social interaction. Ideally, find a setting where these opportunities match with what your loved one enjoys—for example, outdoor versus indoor work, or working with your hands versus intellectual pursuits.

Are outside support structures allowed? If so, how are they accessed?

Understand from the beginning if a setting is self-contained or will allow your provider to continue working with your loved one. Find out if you or the team at the setting will be responsible for adding additional support structures, such as, for example, access to AA or NA meetings.

How much contact does this setting permit with family members?

Seek a setting that believes in maintaining contact with and listening to feedback from family members.

Does this program have the ability to be flexible to accommodate the different phases of healing and recovery for each individual?

Seek a program that is able to recognize your loved one's specific journey, understanding that NBD is complex, and that treatment programs need to be attentive to how residents respond, or not, to psychopharmacological interventions and the social milieu. Ideally, programs understand that while some residents may find a base level of stability after a specific time, others may need a lot longer. When your loved one is in crisis and seriously ill, be wary of programs that advocate for a one-size-fits-all approach.

QUESTIONS TO ASK YOURSELF

Do I feel supported in this journey?

Remind yourself that you need allies. Find a support group, listen to podcasts, read books, and find providers with whom you feel connected and to whom you can turn for encouragement and support. Start with some of the books and podcasts listed in this book in the section following the Appendix.

Do I know enough?

New information is appearing all the time about the biology of NBD and treatment options. Education from articles, books, websites, podcasts, documentaries, and lectures is available and important to access. Never stop asking questions.

How early in the journey should I advocate for a thorough evaluation and sustained treatment for myself or my loved one?

Remind yourself that what has generally been called "mental illness" is actually a brain disease. As with all physical illnesses, early detection and treatment is correlated with better prognosis. The longer the brain succumbs to repeated assault, the more difficult it is and the longer it takes to heal. Early diagnosis and appropriate treatment of psychotic illnesses is very important.

Do I trust my providers?

Remind yourself that trust is a critical variable because achieving long-term stability is a process and can take a long time. Do you feel able to raise anxieties and concerns with your provider? Do you feel there is respect for your perspective, even if they don't agree with it? Having patience in the process is critical, but periodic reevaluation of how the process is going is equally important. A provider should never be condescending or make you feel your questions are invalid. If you are unhappy with your provider, reach out to some of the support groups mentioned in the previous chapter, and you can find recommendations for people in your area.

How much patience should I have for the process of recovery?

Remind yourself that patience is a virtue, but passivity is not. If you trust your providers, let them guide you, but remain an active listener and participant. Remember that psychotic illnesses often involve disorders of development or damage to critical neuroendocrine systems, which are not reset by a simple chemical intervention. Recovery involves cognitive and emotional interventions, and, consequently, improvement and recovery can take many, many months. Don't be afraid to voice your concerns, however. You want to work with a provider who listens to your feelings and works with you and your family.

Do I have reasonable goals?

Remind yourself to let go of early, preconceived expectations about how long the process will take and what the outcome will be. Try to understand what your loved one's or your own current dream may be and then divide recovery goals into shorter-term and longer-term objectives. Don't settle for a stable but isolated existence for yourself or your loved one. Try to understand what a meaningful life would look like at the present moment. Keep advocating for that to be fulfilled.

When should I give up trying if there have been repeated relapses?

Never! But sometimes you need to take a break. This means remembering that you, your partner, and your other children (if you have them), need support, affection, and focus. It is easy to give all your energy to a loved one in crisis and have little left to give the rest of the family. Remind yourself that chronic sacrifice is a problematic equation, because the journey of NBD is lifelong, and you and your family need to refuel. If you don't take active measures to send energy in other directions, you will become depleted, and your family will suffer even more than it has. Challenge yourself to feel joy, even when it is fleeting. Remind yourself about *wabi-sabi* (see Chapter Three).

How should I handle the stigma of NBD?

Remind yourself that people tend to fear and stigmatize things that are foreign because foreign things are easier to simplify, stereotype, and sensationalize. Things are less vulnerable to stigmatization when they are understood, made more personal, and associated with positive outcomes. So those who feel comfortable educating, personalizing, and countering stereotypes about NBD will certainly help in the slow process of changing the perspective about NBD. Some prefer to fight their battles privately, however, understanding that despite slow progress, many still judge people unfairly based on stigma and prejudice. Weigh the risks and benefits of being open about your experience; perhaps the scales will shift at different stages of your journey. If you choose to remain private about your journey, try to find support from people who have lived a similar experience, because being private does not mean you have to be totally isolated. Turning to others when you feel overwhelmed can be part of a healing process.

How should I handle my loved one's anosognosia?

Remind yourself that it is difficult, often impossible, to persuade someone to accept something they don't believe. There may be very complex reasons for your loved one to be in denial. Stay away from focusing on diagnosis. Focus, instead, on addressing specific symptoms in a gentle but persistent fashion. Education about psychiatric illness as a brain disease is important. If your loved one is receptive, provide them with data and research that supports the benefit of medication in controlling uncomfortable symptoms. Align yourself with their desire to get rid of specific uncomfortable issues or attain certain goals. Encourage contact with other patients who accept treatment and are improving. If nothing that you do changes their denial of illness, recognize that you may need to place some boundaries in your relationship during this stage. Take a step back and focus your energy on other things that can reenergize your spirit. Perhaps that takes the form of advocacy, or enjoyment of time with other family members, or engaging in a passion that gives you joy and respite. Acknowledge the sense of loss but accept that there are things beyond your control. (See Chapter Seven for an expanded discussion of anosognosia.)

How should I approach the issue of drug use?

Remind yourself to stay consistent in your message that drug use can be catastrophic for a vulnerable brain, while understanding that we live in a culture that often encourages the use of recreational substances. Arm yourself with data and research that supports this conclusion. If your loved one is using, try to understand what purpose this drug use serves; for example, does it make them feel less anxious and more connected to others? Redirect them to alternative medications or strategies to deal with these issues. As much as is possible, remove them from triggers (such as certain individuals) of drug use. Encourage your loved one to join sober support groups (e.g., AA, NA, Smart Recovery) so that they can have peer support in this process.

How do I remain hopeful?

Connect with providers who believe that an individual with NBD can live a happy life. Connect with some of the resources that are mentioned in these pages and find the ones that work for you. Find a supportive community of people who have had similar experiences and whose willingness to share both their knowledge and emotional journey softens the isolation and loneliness that often accompany this struggle.

STUART'S STORY

I dedicate this piece to all of those who are struggling and may currently find themselves alone in this world without an answer to their problems. I suppose this could be paramount to those who are suffering from some form of mental health ailments, and to those who don't have a viable solution in sight. I must assure you that there is some appropriate pathway of treatment to remedy your mental health challenges in life and that you are not alone. I am a walking and living example of this. Allow me to share my story on how I battled significant mental health issues. Now, after an eighteen-month stint of treatment and recovery at Silver Hill Hospital, under the care of Dr. Marotta and his team, I am 100 percent cured thanks to a medication regimen that now has minimal to no side effects whatsoever.

To those who are lost, and seeking a cure to their mental health issues, I can assure you that you will find your salvation with the proper medication regimen and treatment. I suffered a significant recreational drug overdose, cut with bad substances, in my early twenties that left me with psychosis and auditory hallucinations. Pursuant to this unfortunate event, I had been in and out of mental health clinics from January 2013, all the way to the end of 2022, a ten-year battle with my mental health. I had met with dozens of psychiatrists and had been a part of numerous mental health programs throughout those painfully long-winded years. Many of these doctors put me on SSRIs or antipsychotics, which did not help me as much as I would've hoped. Getting the right combination of medications seemed hopeless. Feeling lost, and without a solution, I bottomed out again in the early part of the pandemic. At that time I was backed into a corner regarding my general mental health and living in a full state of isolation. Soon after, I was referred to Silver Hill Hospital by my psychologist and officially enrolled in the hospital's Michael's House [Lodge] program in March of 2021.

Continued ➤

By reputation Silver Hill is one of the most renowned mental health institutions in the United States. I knew immediately that I was in good hands. At the time of my initial enrollment, my auditory hallucinations, or irrational thinking patterns, were at times very intense. These symptoms were very similar to what I was feeling before I enrolled in Silver Hill's hospital's Michael's House [Lodge] program. Dr. Marotta and Dr. Brown tried a few different medications until they hit on a tremendously effective medication regimen, with Clozapine being the main drug doing the heavy lifting and oxytocin supporting the clozapine. By virtue of the fact that I had a medication liver sensitivity to clozapine, my medication regimen had to slowly be titrated over the course of several months; it required a bit of patience. Knowing this, I had to accept that I would be a patient at Silver Hill Hospital for quite a while.

My time at The Lodge program at Silver Hill was spent learning DBT* skills and coping mechanisms to deal with difficult situations. For example, if I have an intrusive thought around my general health, training my mind to use DBT skills (like check the facts, or opposite action) helped me work through tough situations that I would occasionally deal with.

Eventually, after being at Silver Hill for two months, I hit my groove from a structural/schedule standpoint. I would spend several hours a day listening to a variety of audiobooks, such as biographies or nonfiction books. In addition to that, we had a number of groups or classes run by The Lodge staff. I also spent frequent time in the gym on the cycling machines. Silver Hill does not feel like your typical hospital. It gives off the vibe more synonymous to that of a country club, rather than a hospital. One thing to note, was that I was not as social as I probably should've been. While I was there for eighteen months, most of the other programs aside from The Lodge were four weeks long. As a result, patients cycled in and out of Silver Hill, while I was steadily being treated long-term for several months at The Lodge. I had to accept that I would be a patient at Silver Hill for quite a while.

By reputation, Dr Marotta is considered the best psychiatric doctor in the United States to administer clozapine to his patients. Having previously tried just about every other med regimen, I had my skepticisms. However to the contrary, I adapted well to this new regimen. Not long

* Dialectical Behavior Therapy.

Continued ➤

after, I could feel myself recovering, miraculously having a lucid mindset with minimal to no auditory hallucinations or symptoms like I had suffered for the last decade. My thought patterns were at ease, and I could finally think clearly again. I could not believe that this med regimen built around clozapine had essentially cured my mental health-related problems. My mind was clear and I continued to get stronger day after day. To my disbelief, I was experiencing maximum benefits from clozapine, and literally minimal to no side effects. I was absolutely amazed by how effective this medication regimen was, and as a result it has dramatically improved the quality of my life. I may even go as far to say that this med regimen saved my life in some regard. Now here I am eighteen months after being discharged from Dr. Marotta's and Dr. Brown's care, and from Silver Hill, and I have to say that my mental health is as good as it's ever been before. Many thanks to Dr. Marotta, Dr. Brown, and the whole team at Silver Hill. I am feeling rejuvenated, ready to take on the world, and as good as new!

My time at Silver Hill was the most profound experience regarding my mental health, considering that I had been treated for my mental health on and off over the course of a ten-year period. I would say now in April of 2024, I continue to improve and get better and better. Having this steady team around me has given me the opportunity to thrive, and I feel better than ever as a result.

Epilogue by Dr. Rocco Marotta:
Finding True North and Future Directions

When Drs. Mann and Dougherty asked me to write an epilogue to their book describing the work of our team over the last fifteen years or so at Silver Hill Hospital, my first attempt consisted of a narrative of the problems posed to us in trying to treat severe psychiatric illness in young adults. There were so many points of frustration exacting a great toll of misery in our patients and their families, who, out of love and sheer will, persisted in searching for help. So many of them feared for the lives of their children and families, and there were years of confusing advice, self-doubt, and exhausting struggle. There were the emotional and financial costs to all involved, including society and the health-care systems.

I outlined that trying to understand our failures, my own and the system we serve, ultimately helped us to recognize that we had a powerful intervention, clozapine, which, while not perfect, was a superior medication overall for the treatment of resistant psychotic illnesses, especially in our setting at The Lodge, where we were caring for so many patients who had had so many unsuccessful previous treatment trials. Increasing use of clozapine, which posed its own technical and administrative issues, led to placing more emphasis on the mitigation of side effects, and the use of more complex medication regimens led us to new problems, new interventions, more problems, and yet still successes. I tried to outline this and give data and the flow of therapeutic reasoning: clozapine, to the addition of oxytocin, to the addition of Lamictal, to trials of procholinergic medications, to weight control interventions, gym visits and cooking groups, and family programs, etc., showing overall improvement in patient outcome, all ending in a justification for not running double-blind placebo control studies, since we could clearly see that patients were improving. They went to school, they had jobs, they were sober and compliant, and many were actually happy. While applauding my efforts, Drs. Mann and Dougherty sent me back to the drawing board. "Be less academic, more personal," they said.

I promise to do so but ask for a little more indulgence for my musings. Over the years, our team has rededicated itself to the old imperatives of medicine: while doing no harm, our aim should be more than just the alleviation of "target" symptoms, more than being able to assert on a discharge note that over the next seventy-two hours "this young man will not be an acute danger to himself or others and will be able to feed himself and find shelter." Years ago, we began to embrace the idea that our patients, like us, deserved a chance at some happiness and even success beyond the absence of command auditory hallucinations, and that their families deserved some relief from the PTSD and guilt induced by the constant fears for the safety and well-being of their children. To continue with our book's metaphor, we wanted to mend the lines and sheets and caulk the hulls and sails of each vessel, so that the voyage could be continued and the storms and challenges of life endured. Our target is not the lowering of PANSS ratings to attain a statistically significant quantitative result, but to get our patients back to sea—for example, back to and through school (some have earned master's and beyond), working, and having relationships with friends and family. It is heartening, for example, that Eliot remembered to get his mother a birthday present!

The team and I are not alone in our desire for a different outcome for our patients with NBD. The vast majority of mental health practitioners share these hopes. Most began their careers motivated by the desire to help others, but in my experience, many are now frustrated (or burnt out) by a system that does not seem to work well in the delivery of care to the most ill psychiatric patients, a society unable to effectively address the consequence of substance use, and the breakdown of family and community support systems. We see in our society's struggle to deal with the problem of homelessness a consequence of our inability to successfully address the continuing epidemic of NBD. Luckily, we are working at Silver Hill Hospital, an institution that affords us the material, emotional, and intellectual support to try new things and to fight to hold patients longer. We are also most blessed to have the support of so many families who trust us to work with their children for extended periods of time so that we can create detailed and individualized treatment plans and follow a large number of Lodge graduates for years. We are also so lucky to have partners in outside agencies and programs (for example, Spring Lake Ranch, Gould Farm, CooperRiis, Partners Creating Community, The Dorm) that we can refer to. We even have the dedication of individuals like Paul Demirjian, who started his own program, Safe Harbors, to give support to our discharged patients. It is important to be able to work with others who share our views, like Drs. Laitman and Mandel, who embrace the use of clozapine as a primary medication. This is critical, since we, and others, have had the unfortunate experience of tragic outcomes when patients have been taken off of clozapine by other groups. That patients suffering from NBD be afforded compassionate and effective care is a matter of equity, and to not do so is to place hundreds of thousands of our fellow citizens at risk of suffering unnecessarily.

Drs. Mann and Dougherty have been patient with me, so now let me tell you how I got to this place in the pilgrimage that is my life. I was lucky to be raised in a loving home, with a large, boisterous, extended family. They cared for each other in complex and continuous ways. Almost any idiosyncrasy was tolerated, all was ultimately forgiven, and there was always a woman, a special "Aunt," with unspoken powers, who was there to listen and calm the disturbances. In my intergenerational amalgam of clans, my own mother was the special "Aunt," the quiet one, keeper of secrets, who was the recognized and consulted one. She had the secret stigmata and gifts of a Mediterranean sibyl—one blue eye and one green, for example—but her power and skill came from listening nonjudgmentally and loving unconditionally. I, for one, thought she could read my mind! And then, of course, the men, with their example of stoic acceptance that struggle is inherent to life and caring for others their duty. The effect of my parents' love was reinforced and focused by my teachers, who were often nuns, brothers, and priests who dedicated their lives to the care of others. They set a very high standard of idealism and commitment. And I have been blessed to work in a setting with a team that would, deservedly, garner their praise.

When my willingness to enter the army in the summer of 1970 was blocked by an unexpected or unsought deferral, I was at first unaware that the "Spirit of the Great Mothers," beautifully depicted in the mosaics in the Cathedral in Siena, were simply bending fate to move me to where they knew I was meant to be—not a soldier, but an *iatos*, a healer, with a different kind of "life in the trenches," as our Lodge team calls it. So, instead of twelve weeks at Fort Dix, I went to twelve years of training at the City University of New York, Cornell Medical College, and the New York Hospital. There was a lot to learn. I have been lucky to spend my life doing something I love, and lucky to work with colleagues whose passion for helping others is deeply rooted. I wish for everyone this kind of passion. The fates had other ways to teach me as well. One of our children struggles with bipolar illness. I was already involved in a life dedicated to the treatment of this type of disease when parenthood brought me a new dimension of understanding. As those of you who are parents of children with NBD all know, lived experience is humbling and requires courage.

Even with support, it is difficult to do this work. At dinner the other night, a young colleague asked me, "Do you think that psychiatry as we practice it at The Lodge can survive in our modern culture of digitized and insurance-driven medical care?" In other words, can an approach that requires patience and is predicated on relationships continue, let alone flourish, in a world that pushes compartmentalized services and quick fixes? I think the honest answer is that the medical profession is an intrinsically altruistic one, but it is easy to lose sight of the bigger picture. The norm is now increasing specialization and the entrance of corporate values leading to the emptying of hospital beds and the assembly line of outpatient care with checklist treatment plans. We need leaders who will fight the battle to maintain a different perspective, who will ask the question about each patient, "What is our objective?", and will give the answer "to save this person and this soul," not "to get them out as quickly as possible." At The Lodge we believe this can only be accomplished by helping patients regain a sense of who they want to be. Medication and technology are not sufficient for this task. It takes treatment which mingles the scientific and measurable with the instinctive and ephemeral. It takes professionals who are willing to share their humanity by opening themselves up to connecting, loving, inspiring, both with each other and with their patients. It involves standing up for what you feel is right, not necessarily "correct." It involves daring to create a different choreography, and hopefully inspiring others to join the dance.

My hope for the future is that The Lodge program at SHH will continue to serve its patients under the care of its dedicated staff, to treat each patient as an individual who needs their guidance and concern on many levels; that the team continues to have the leave to slowly and gently address the anosognosia (denial of illness) and paranoia of our patients, not as flaws in their character but as intrinsic aspects of a disorder to be overcome through understanding and medical care. It is my hope that with mentorship, it will be some of the younger doctors in our society who take up the battle and, while embracing new advances in medicine, do not lose sight of the person behind the diagnosis. In the inimitable words of Carl Jung, "Know all the theories, master all the techniques, but as you touch a human soul be just another human soul." Teamwork, alliances with different medical disciplines and the field of criminal justice, and the sharing of knowledge is at the heart of change. We recognize how difficult this journey is, but my vision is this:

> That we all remain clear in our objectives and responsibilities.
> That we remember our task: *cura animae*, the healing of souls
> and the saving of lives.
> We may rest.
> We may retreat.
> We may even be forced to attack in reverse, but we never give up.
> We use science.
> We practice the art.

We are here to place at the disposal of all who come to us all the knowledge and skills that have been passed on to us by our teachers and colleagues. The work is hard, the journey long, and the "weather" too often uncertain. But then there are those moments of breathtaking beauty and transformation, when you see why you undertook this journey in the first place, and you know that it is all worth it.

> *Everyone's voice was suddenly lifted;*
> *And beauty came like the setting sun;*
> *My heart was shaken with tears; and horror*
> *Drifted away ... O, but Everyone*
> *Was a bird; and the song was wordless; the singing will never be done.*
> —Siegfried Sassoon, from "Everyone Sang," 1919

—Rocky

Postscript

Time marches on. During the course of writing this book, Dr. Marotta transitioned from his role as clinical director of The Lodge program, focusing his time on the directorship of The Center for the Treatment and Study of Neuropsychiatric Disorders. In this role he continues to consult, teach, and mentor The Lodge staff but is also involved with research and educational initiatives. Some of the team members referenced in this book have also transitioned to other jobs since the writing of this book began. The Lodge team continues to focus on helping its patients find fulfilling lives and sustain their recoveries.

ACKNOWLEDGMENTS

This book would not have been possible without the support and funding of the Center for the Treatment and Study of Neuropsychiatric Disorders at Silver Hill Hospital. The authors would also like to acknowledge the support and encouragement of Dr. Andrew Gerber, President and Medical Director of Silver Hill Hospital, whose belief in the project has been steadfast.

We are deeply indebted to the staff of the Lodge Program, former patients and family members, and, above all, to Dr. Marotta. Their generous contributions are the foundation upon which this book was written. We are also grateful to Randye Kaye and Ana Cutts Dougherty whose reading of early drafts provided important feedback. Finally, a heartfelt thank you to Lisa Akoury-Ross, Kent Sorsky, Beth Raps, Gina Sartirana, and Howard Johnson at SDP Publishing.

ENDNOTES

INTRODUCTION

1. Thomas Insel, MD, *Healing: Our Path from Mental Illness to Mental Health* (Penguin Press, 2022), xv–xvi.

2. 2022 data from the Department of Health and Human Services' Mental and Substance Use Disorders Prevalence Study (MSDP) are found in *Profiles in Mental Health Courage*, by Patrick J. Kennedy and Stephen Fried (Penguin Random House, 2024), 13.

3. Sonya C. Faber, et al., "The weaponization of medicine: Early psychosis in the Black community and the need for racially informed mental healthcare." *Frontiers in Psychiatry* 14:1098292.

CHAPTER THREE

1. "Japanese Culture: The Actual Meaning of Wabi-Sabi," Nakamoto Forestry, published October 2021.

2. Pauline Boss, *Ambiguous Loss: Learning to Live with Unresolved Grief* (Harvard University Press, 1999).

CHAPTER FOUR

1. C. U. Correll et al., "A Guideline and Checklist for Initiating and Managing Clozapine Treatment in Patients with Treatment-Resistant Schizophrenia," *CNS Drugs* 36, no. 7, (2022): 659-679.

2. The Warrior Moms support group, joined by the first set of parents from SHH, was curated by Virgil Stucker, who brought together ten mothers from around the US to provide self-guided support for each other. Since their founding, there are now three Warrior Moms groups in existence, each with ten participants. Like the Warrior Moms groups, there are now a growing number of other groups connecting alumni mothers from The Lodge, allowing them to share their stories and lift one another up as they continue to support their loved ones. Other support groups involving alumni caregivers outside of SHH include Angry Moms, a group founded to lobby and advocate for the safe use of clozapine for their loved ones. The Angry Moms' mission to dismantle the current

clozapine Risk Evaluation and Mitigation Strategy and transfer oversight to prescribing physicians, who can enforce rational guidelines for the safe use of clozapine, has recently been successful. Virgil Stucker's website is https://stuckersmithweatherly.com/.

CHAPTER FIVE

1. W. W. Meissner, "The Concept of the Therapeutic Alliance," *Journal of the American Psychoanalytic Association* 40, no. 4 (1992): 1059-87.

2. T. Clifford Allbutt, *Greek Medicine in Rome*, (Macmillan and Co., Limited, 1921), 288-299.

3. Oliver Sacks, "The Lost Virtues of the Asylum," *New York Review of Books*, Sept. 24, 2009.

4. S. Leucht, et al., "60 Years of Placebo-Controlled Antipsychotic Drug Trials in Acute Schizophrenia: Meta-Regression of Predictors of Placebo Response," *Schizophrenia Research* 201 (2018): 315-23.

5. D. Naber and M. Lambert, "The CATIE and CUTLASS studies in schizophrenia: results and implications for clinicians," *CNS Drugs* 23, no. 8 (2009): 649-59.

6. D. Myran et al., "Association Between Non-Medical Cannabis Legalization and Emergency Department Visits for Cannabis-Induced Psychosis," *Mol Psychiatry* 28, no. 10 (2023): 4251-60.

7. Rocco Marotta, MD, PhD, interview with authors, March 19, 2023.

CHAPTER SEVEN

1. Bethany Yeiser, BS and Henry A. Nasrallah, MD, *Awakenings: Stories of Recovery and Emergence from Schizophrenia* (Bethany Yeiser, 2024). This book includes a compilation of stories about successful emergence from a diagnosis of schizophrenia.

2. Jeffrey A. Lieberman, MD, *Malady of the Mind: Schizophrenia and the Path to Prevention* (Scribner 2023), 141-48.

3. Elyn Saks, "Some Thoughts on Denial of Mental Illness," *Am J Psychiatry* 166, no. 9 (2009).

4. Paul Lysaker et al., "The Role of Insight in the Process of Recovery from Schizophrenia: A Review of Three Views," *Psychosis*, no 1 (2009): 113-21.

5. K. J. McKenzie, "How Does Untreated Psychosis Lead to Neurological Damage?," *Canadian Journal of Psychiatry* 59, no. 10 (2014): 511–2.

6. D. Lin et al., "Associations Between Relapses and Psychosocial Outcomes in Patients With Schizophrenia in Real-World Settings in the United States," *Frontiers in Psychiatry* 12 (2021).

7. J. Y. Khokhar et al., "The Link Between Schizophrenia and Substance Use Disorder: A Unifying Hypothesis," *Schizophrenia Research* 194 (2018): 78–85.

8. M. Luciano et al., "Editorial: Mortality of People with Severe Mental Illness: Causes and Ways of its Reduction, *Frontiers in Psychiatry* 13 (2022).

9. Laura Brancato, JD, interview with authors, June 26, 2024.

10. Ibid.

11. Ibid.

12. "Luigi Mangione, Jordan Neely: Mental Illness in the News? One Mother's Opinion." Randye Kaye.com, published December 14, 2024.

CHAPTER EIGHT

1. Paraphrased from the Spring Lake Ranch website, accessed February 20, 2025, https://www.springlakeranch.org.

2. NAMI website, accessed February 20, 2025, https://www.nami.org.

Appendix

The following are publications, presentations, and research collaborations connected to The Center for the Treatment and Study of Neuropsychiatric Disorders (CTSND), directed by Dr. Rocco Marotta.

Publications

Garakani, Amir, Frank D. Buono, and Rocco F. Marotta. "Sublingual Oxytocin With Clozapine in a Patient With Persisting Psychotic Symptoms, Suicidal Thinking With Self-Harm." *J Clin Psychopharmacology* 40, no. 5 (2020): 507–509.

Marotta, Rocco F., Frank D. Buono, Amir Garakani, et al. "The Effects of Augmenting Clozapine with Oxytocin in Schizophrenia: An Initial Case Series." *Annals of Clinical Psychiatry* 32, no. 2 (2020): 90–96.

Marotta, Rocco F., Frank Buono, Amir Garakani, et al. "T198. Can Augmented Sublingual Oxytocin Decrease Negative Symptoms Within Treatment Resistant Schizophrenic Populations: A Pilot Study." *Schizophrenia Bulletin* 46, Suppl 1 (2020): S307.

Marotta, Rocco F., David Rowe, Eric Collins, et al. "F108. Concurrent Usage Of Sublingual Oxytocin And Clozapine To Treat The Positive And Negative Symptoms Within Individuals With Treatment-Resistant Schizophrenia." *Schizophrenia Bulletin* 45, Suppl 2, (2019): S294-S295.

Presentations

Marotta, Rocco F., "Onset of Illness: the Changing Face of Severe Psychiatric Illness in the Early 21st Century." Oral presentation at the Center for the Treatment and Study of Neuropsychiatric Disorders, Silver Hill Hospital, Grace Farms Conference, The Long Course of Care: Interfaces of Multiple Systems and Stakeholders, December 2024.

Marotta, Rocco F., "Cannabis and Stimulants: Unraveling Psychosis and Novel Clinical Presentation." Oral presentation at The Dorm Webinar, November 2024.

Marotta, Rocco F., Lisa Mann, Katharine Cutts Dougherty, et. al. "Expanding Directions in the Treatment of Serious Mental Illness: Beyond the Double Blind," Paper presented at The Center for the Treatment and Study of Neuropsychiatric Disorders Colloquium, Rome, Italy, April 2024.

Marotta, Rocco F., Irene Bihl, Meriwether Brown, et al. "Building a Continuum of Care for Treatment-Resistant Schizophrenia Spectrum Disorders." Poster presented at the Congress of the Schizophrenia International Research Society, April 2024.

Walker, Sophia, Katharine Cutts Dougherty, Howard Weiner, et al. "Complex Seizure Disorder Symptoms Manifesting in Treatment-Resistant Schizophrenia Spectrum Disorders in Young Adults with Prior Cannabis Use: A Clinical Overview." Poster presented at the Congress of the Schizophrenia International Research Society, April 2024.

Marotta, Rocco F., "Treatment-Resistant Schizophrenia in Young Adulthood: Treatment Strategies and Common Barriers," Virtual Continuing Education Presentation at The Dorm, November 2023.

Marotta, Rocco F., "Neuropsychiatric Manifestations of COVID Infections: Clinical Presentations & Possible Underlying Pathophysiology." Oral presentation at Silver Hill Hospital Virtual Grand Rounds, June 2023.

Marotta, Rocco F., Katharine Cutts Dougherty, Meriwether Brown, et al. "Maximizing Recovery from Schizophrenia Spectrum Disorders in a Hospital/Residential Setting: Clozapine, Oxytocin, Psychosocial and Family Programs." Poster presented at the American Psychiatric Association Annual Meeting, May 2023.

Rocco F. Marotta, Katharine Cutts Dougherty, Frank Buono, et al. "Long-Term Effects of Clozapine and Oxytocin on Functional Recovery and Sobriety Maintenance in Treatment Resistant Schizophrenia." Oral presentation to the Congress of the Schizophrenia International Research Society, April 2022.

Marotta, Rocco F., "Addressing the Common Course of Schizophrenia: Effect of Clozapine and Sublingual Oxytocin on Substance Use Relapse and Long-Term Life Trajectories." Paper presented to the American Academy of Addiction Psychiatry Annual Meeting and Scientific Symposium, December 2021.

Marotta, Rocco F., "Oxytocin as an Augmentation to the Treatment of Schizophrenia with Clozapine: Improvement in Negative Symptoms and Life Paths." Oral presentation to New York-Presbyterian Westchester Hospital, May 2021.

Rocco F. Marotta, "Oxytocin as an Augmentation to the Treatment of Schizophrenia with Clozapine: Improvement in Negative Symptoms and Life Paths." Oral presentation at Silver Hill Hospital Grand Rounds, March 2021.

Marotta, Rocco F., "Oxytocin as an Augmentation to the Treatment of Schizophrenia with Clozapine: Improvement in Negative Symptoms and

Life Paths." Oral presentation at Institute of Living, Hartford Hospital Grand Rounds, January 2021.

Marotta, Rocco F., Katharine Cutts Dougherty, David Rowe, et al. "Can Augmented Sublingual Oxytocin Decrease Negative Symptoms within Treatment Resistant Schizophrenic Populations: A Pilot Study." Poster presented at the Congress of the Schizophrenia International Research Society, April 2020.

Marotta, Rocco F., "Creative Psychiatry: Learn about the Benefits of Oxytocin for Psychosis." Interview by Virgil Stucker. *Mental Horizons, S3EP3,* https:// podcasts.apple.com/us/podcast/s3ep3-creative-psychiatry-with-rocco-marotta-learn/id1476557069?i=1000492480387

Dr. Marotta and his team conducted a monthly Neuropsychiatric Case Conference Program for Silver Hill Hospital clinicians. This program increased clinical understanding of treating patients with persistent psychotic illness, especially those who had undergone multiple unsuccessful interventions.

RESEARCH COLLABORATIONS

Mercedes Perez-Rodriguez, MD, PhD, Mount Sinai Hospital
The Center for the Treatment and Study of Neuropsychiatric Disorders has funded a collaboration with Dr. Perez-Rodriguez to study the absorption of sublingual oxytocin in the bloodstream. Approved by the Mount Sinai Institutional Review Board, this study has begun enrolling participants.

Michael McGee, MD, Atascadero State Hospital
Dr. Marotta and the CTSND have been collaborating with Dr. McGee, a Distinguished Life Fellow of the American Psychiatric Association, to conduct a feasibility study about the impact of oxytocin on this forensic hospital's patients who have been stabilized on clozapine. The study was designed to explore whether adding sublingual oxytocin to patients' medication regimes would increase their overall psychosocial functioning, allowing a higher percentage of patients to return to community life. While the study protocol was approved by the CA State Medical Review Board, sadly it has not been allowed to run by state hospital authorities. Other collaborations are ongoing.

Sage Healthcare Clinic is an academically supported organization that strives to provide best practices in a holistic care environment, including family practice, behavioral and mental health, social work, and case management. This clinic is attached to Bridgeport Rescue Mission, in Bridgeport, Connecticut. Dr. Marotta serves as the Medical Director, Behavioral Health. Research program is in the process of being developed.

DATA SPECIFIC TO THE ISSUE OF SOBRIETY AND PSYCHOTIC ILLNESS

- Review of patient data at SHH by the neuropsychiatric team revealed that eighty percent of young people admitted and treated for severe psychotic disorders had histories of exposure to cannabis and stimulants. These cases appeared more floridly ill and harder to treat.

- Our experience and that of other clinical teams has been confirmed and extended by data from Scandinavia which shows an increase in the rates of schizophrenia in Finland and Denmark. The Danish data clearly show a marked effect which correlates with the availability of high potency cannabis.

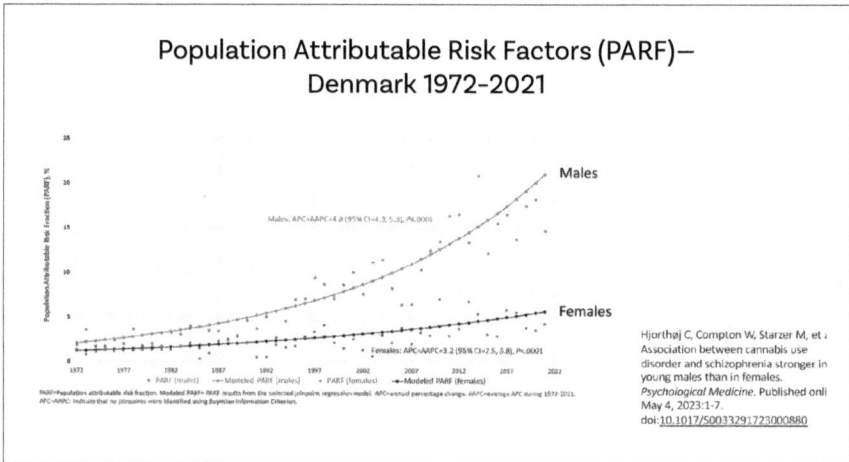

FIGURE 6: *Population Attributable Risk Factors (PARF)—Denmark 1972—2021*

This image shows the result of statistical analysis of Danish data, revealing that the increased risk of developing schizophrenia was due to cannabis and not other factors such as social class, other drugs, educational level, or family history. In fact, researchers estimated that twenty-five percent of cases of schizophrenia diagnosed in Denmark could have been prevented by decreased use of cannabis.

Source: Slide presented at Silver Hill Hospital Grace Farms conference, December 2024, reference on slide.

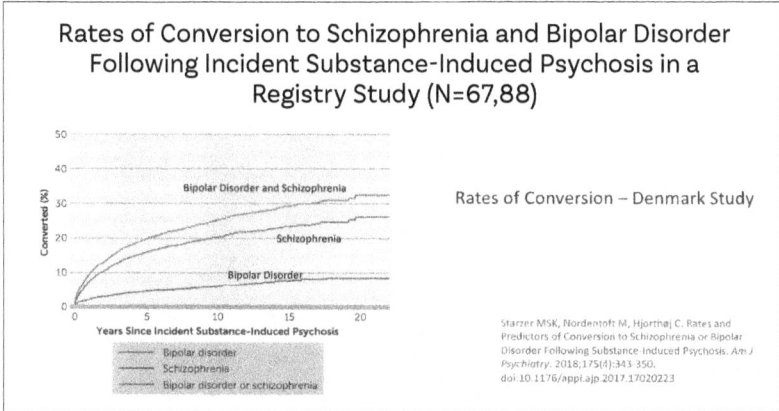

FIGURE 7: *Rates of Conversion to Schizophrenia and Bipolar Disorder Following Incident Substance-Induced Psychosis in a Registry Study (N=67,88).*

This image illustrates that if a person has had a psychotic reaction to cannabis that needs medical attention, the risk of that person eventually being diagnosed as suffering from schizophrenia over the next years was very high—thirty percent more than expected.

Source: Slide presented at Silver Hill Hospital Grace Farms conference, December 2024, reference on slide.

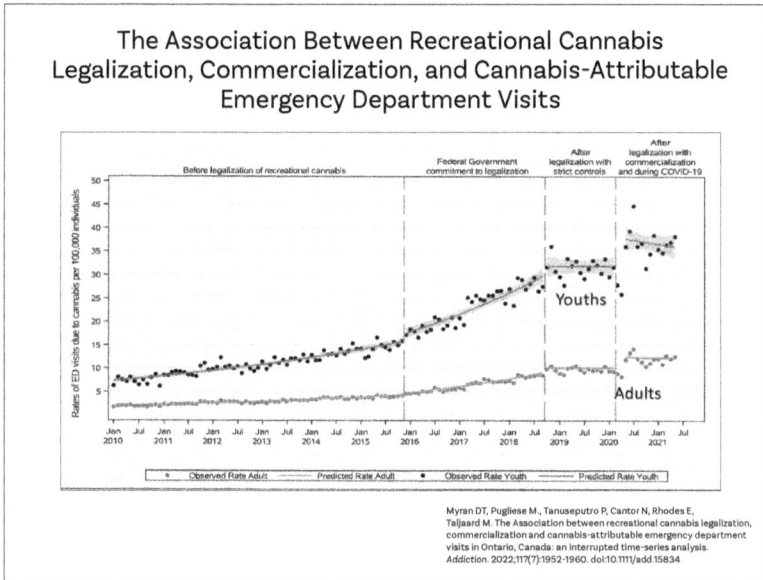

FIGURE 8: *The Association Between Recreational Cannabis Legalization, Commercialization, and Cannabis-Attributable Emergency Department Visits in Ontario*

Data from Ontario, Canada confirms the increase in incidence of psychosis and diagnosis of schizophrenia over the last years and shows that emergency room visits have increased remarkably with increasing availability of cannabis and the social acceptance of its use.

Source: Slide presented at Silver Hill Hospital Grace Farms conference, December 2024, reference on slide.

RECOMMENDED RESOURCES

These recommendations are by no means exhaustive. They are examples of books and podcasts that we feel provide both information and support for families on the NBD journey.

PODCAST

The podcast *Schizophrenia: Three Moms in the Trenches* is hosted by Randye Kaye, Mindy Greiling, and Miriam Feldman, three mothers whose sons have been diagnosed with schizophrenia. The hosts, each of whom has written a book about their experiences, deal with a wide range of topics and personal stories in a conversational, interview format. They also provide extensive resource lists and links for their listeners and readers.

PERSONAL STORIES

Awakenings: Stories of Recovery and Emergence from Schizophrenia, by Bethany Yeiser, BS, and Henry A. Nasrallah, MD.

Ben Behind His Voices: One Family's Journey from the Chaos of Schizophrenia to Hope, by Randye Kaye.

Crazy: A Father's Search Through America's Mental Health Madness, by Pete Earley.

Fix What You Can: Schizophrenia and a Lawmaker's Fight for Her Son, by Mindy Greiling.

He Came in With It: A Portrait of Motherhood and Madness, by Miriam Feldman.

Meaningful Recovery from Schizophrenia and Serious Mental Illness with Clozapine, by Lewis Opler, MD, Robert Laitman, MD, Ann Mandel Laitman, MD, and Daniel Laitman.

Profiles in Mental Health Courage, curated and annotated by Patrick J. Kennedy and Stephen Fried.

The Best Minds: A Story of Friendship, Madness, and the Tragedy of Good Intentions, by Jonathan Rosen.

The Center Cannot Hold: My Journey Through Madness, by Elyn R. Saks.

The Quiet Room: A Journey out of the Torment of Madness, by Lori Schiller and Amanda Bennett.

OVERVIEWS OF SCHIZOPHRENIA AND RELATED DISORDERS AND INFORMATIONAL GUIDES

A Family Guide to Mental Health Recovery: What You Need to Know from Day One, by Virgil Stucker and Stephanie McMahon.

I Am Not Sick I Don't Need Help!: How to Help Someone Accept Treatment, by Xavier Amador, PhD.

Healing: Our Path from Mental Illness to Mental Health, by Thomas Insel, MD.

Loving Someone with a Mental Illness or History of Trauma: Skills, Hope, and Strength for Your Journey, by Michelle D. Sherman, PhD, ABPP, and DeAnne M. Sherman.

Malady of the Mind: Schizophrenia and the Path to Prevention, by Jeffrey A. Lieberman, MD.

Schizophrenia & Related Disorders: A Handbook for Caregivers, by Nicole Drapeau Gillen.

Surviving Schizophrenia: a Family Manual, Seventh Edition, by E. Fuller Torrey, MD.

The Clozapine Handbook, by Jonathan M. Meyer, MD and Stephen M. Stahl, MD, PhD.

ABOUT THE AUTHORS

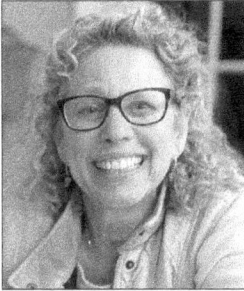

LISA MANN, PhD, is a clinical psychologist, educated at Harvard University, New York University, and St. Luke's/Roosevelt Hospital Center in New York City. Licensed in both New York and Connecticut, during the past four decades, Dr. Mann has been involved in both teaching and clinical practice, directing the Training and Psychological Services, Division of Child and Adolescent Psychiatry at St. Luke's/Roosevelt Hospital Center from 1992–1996, working as a lower school division psychologist at the Trinity School in New York City from 1996–2000, and seeing children and adults in her personal clinical practice. Her interest in the world of neuropsychiatric brain disease comes from both personal and professional experiences, and she is a passionate advocate of parent education in the field of mental health. Dr. Mann has always enjoyed writing. Her first book project was the posthumous compilation and editing of writings of her father, Robert Mann, the founder of the Juilliard String Quartet (*A Passionate Journey: a Memoir*). Collaborating with Katharine Cutts Dougherty, PhD, on *Lives Reimagined: Changing the Course of Psychotic Illness*, and working closely with the courageous patients, families, and staff who have dedicated their lives to this issue, has been an exciting and inspiring experience. Married to Rocco F. Marotta, MD, PhD, the director of The Center for the Treatment and Study of Serious Neuropsychiatric Disorders, the topic is never far from her mind. In her free time, however, Dr. Mann enjoys her three children and their spouses, and her two grandchildren, who light up her life. Dr. Mann is also an avid ballet dancer and knitter. She resides in both Ridgefield, CT, and Charleston, SC.

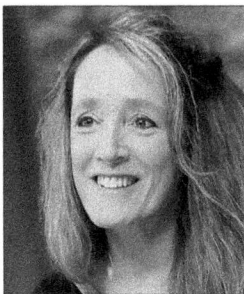

KATHARINE CUTTS DOUGHERTY, PhD, worked as the Senior Research Associate to Dr. Rocco Marotta at the Center for the Study and Treatment of Neuropsychiatric Disorders at Silver Hill Hospital in New Canaan, Connecticut from 2019-2024. With a strong personal and professional interest in education and mental health, and as a "trailing spouse," she has woven a career across states and continents over the past three decades. Educated in South Africa, Argentina, England, and the US, she earned a First-Class BA degree in Psychology from Exeter University, UK, a MS in Human Development and Family Studies from Cornell University, US, and a PhD in Education from the

University of Colorado at Boulder, US. Among many roles, she has worked as an ethnographer on a National Child Development Program, an examiner for the psychology portion of the International Baccalaureate Program, a Visiting Professor in the Department of Education at Dartmouth College, and the Director of Community and Global Citizenship at Albuquerque Academy. She currently has a private practice as a certified life coach. Along with many of those who will read this book, her "professional" career has most often taken a second seat to a primary role as a caregiver providing stability and support for family and loved ones.

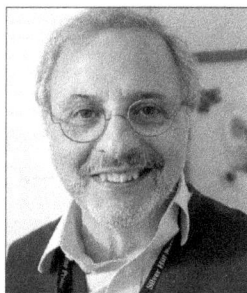

Rocco F. Marotta, MD, PhD, Director, Center for the Treatment and Study of Neuropsychiatric Disorders and founder of The Lodge Program, Silver Hill Hospital, in New Canaan, CT, began his interest in psychiatric treatment as a young man, working as a psychiatric aide in a big city hospital during the years of the early lithium trials. Fascinated by the remarkable positive change lithium made in patients' psychiatric states, he decided to pursue his PhD in Biology and Neuropsychology at City University of New York, with a specialized interest in the biology behind brain behavior. An avid teacher, he worked as an assistant professor at both Mount Saint Vincent and Hunter College, also teaching medical students about the biology of the brain. His research, focused on facilitating recovery from brain trauma using psychopharmacologic agents, eventually won him a fellowship at Montefiore Hospital in the Bronx, NY, under the leadership of the inspiring physician Herbert Weiner, MD.

Encouraged by his wife and supported by Dr. Weiner's belief in his candidacy, Dr. Marotta applied to medical school at the ripe old age of 33 years, a decade older than most of the medical students who would be his peers. He attended Cornell Medical School, doing his residency in psychiatry at Payne Whitney Clinic at New York Hospital and continuing his interest in both medication management and clinical treatment of psychotic illness. Dr. Marotta's professional life has included roles as Director of Danbury Hospital's Inpatient Psychiatric Services, Service Chief of the Medical Psychiatric Unit at Westchester Medical Center, Department of Psychiatry and Behavioral Science, and Service Chief of Silver Hill's Transitional Living Program, during which time he started The Lodge Program. While his professional affiliations have shifted during his decades-long practice of psychiatry, his love of teaching and collaboration with colleagues has been steadfast. Dr. Marotta's belief in the power of relationship in treatment is present in all that he does.

Dr. Marotta, or Rocky, as he is known to all, has been married for forty-four years to Lisa Mann, PhD, coauthor of this book. They have three children and two grandchildren, and split their time between Ridgefield, Connecticut, and Charleston, South Carolina.

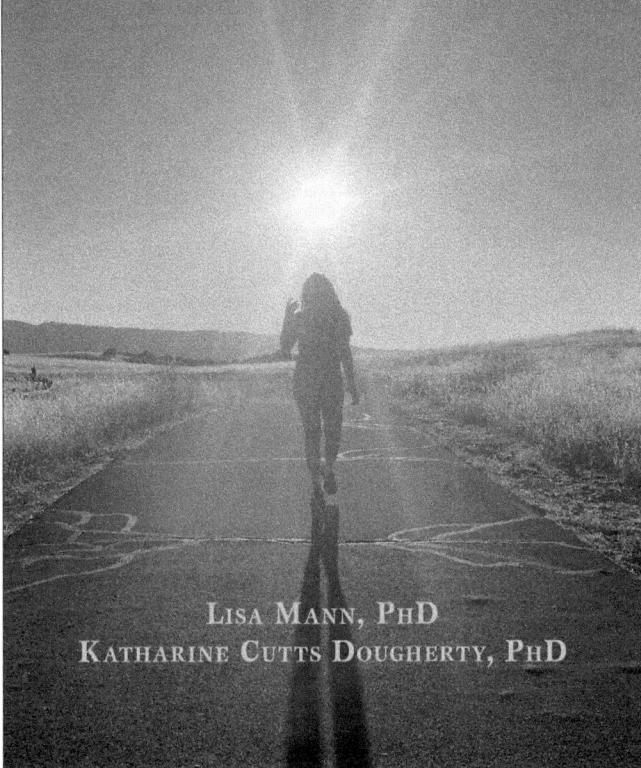

Lives Reimagined

Changing the Course of Psychotic Illness

Lisa Mann, PhD
Katharine Cutts Dougherty, PhD

Also available in ebook format

SDP Publishing

www.SDPPublishing.com

Contact us at: info@SDPPublishing.com